Textbook of Medical Statistics

Xiuhua Guo • Fuzhong Xue

Editors

Textbook of Medical Statistics

For Medical Students

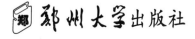 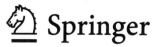

Editors
Xiuhua Guo
School of public health
Capital Medical University
Beijing, China

Fuzhong Xue
School of Public Health
Shandong University
Jinan, China

ISBN 978-981-99-7389-7   ISBN 978-981-99-7390-3   (eBook)
https://doi.org/10.1007/978-981-99-7390-3

Contents

Chapter 1
Introduction to Medical Statistics

Fuzhong Xue, Tong Wang, and Shicheng Yu

> **Objectives**
> Statistics is the science of collecting, analyzing, and interpreting data. The objective of this chapter is to introduce basic statistical concepts, such as variables, types of data, probability, populations, and samples. Students should also understand the steps of statistical work after studying this chapter.

> **Key Concepts**
> Quantitative and qualitative data; continuous and discrete variables; ordinal and categorical variables; probability; populations and samples; parameters and statistics.

1.1 The Definition of Medical Statistics

Medical statistics plays a key role in medical research, evidence-based medicine, evidence-based public health policy-making, etc. In medical research, data must be collected and analyzed in order to answer a specific research question. During this

F. Xue (✉)
School of Public Health, Shandong University, Jinan, China
e-mail: xuefzh@sdu.edu.cn

T. Wang
School of Public Health, Shandong University, Taiyuan, China

S. Yu
National Center for Public Health Surveillance and Information Services, Chinese Center for Disease Control and Prevention, Beijing, China

© Zhengzhou University Press 2024   1
X. Guo, F. Xue (eds.), *Textbook of Medical Statistics*,
https://doi.org/10.1007/978-981-99-7390-3_1

process, medical statistics provides knowledge of the study design, data collection, data management, data analysis, and interpretation of the results. Before a new drug, treatment, or device can be marketed, an experimental study or quasi-experimental study must be conducted to evaluate the effectiveness and safety of the new health technique and service. In addition, many other questions need to be addressed. What major health problems are currently present in the region? From where do increases in healthcare spending originate? Where should a government invest its resources if it wishes to reduce the rate of birth defects? What are the effects of workplace health and safety on the nurses' employment rates? What types of services are used by long-term homecare users, and how has this service changed over time? What factors are associated with the increased risk of ischemic heart disease (IHD)? To answer these questions and many others, methods and skills of medical statistics are essential. Most importantly, researchers can inform policy-makers and influence public health policy-making with evidence from the research, analysis, data series, and evaluation, in which medical statistics plays an important role.

Statistics is the science of collecting, organizing, analyzing, and interpreting numerical facts that we call data. It also involves planning a study in terms of principles of the study design, such as surveys and experiments. Biostatistics is the application of statistics to a wide range of topics in biology. The science of biostatistics involves (1) the design of biological experiments, especially in medicine and agriculture; (2) the collection, summarization, and analysis of data from those experiments; and (3) the interpretation of, and inference from, the results. As opposed to biostatistics, medical statistics involves applications of statistics to medicine and health sciences, including epidemiology, public health, forensic medicine, and clinical research. Simply, medical statistics is the practice of statistics in medical sciences.

1.2 Variables and Types of Data

A set of numbers, composed of data manipulated to obtain an average or a graph, provides insight into the data. To do so, classifying data and identifying types of data are essential for thoroughly understanding the context of data.

A variable is a characteristic of interest about each individual element. Variables could be weight, age, blood pressure, or occupation, and many other things. Variables can be classified as either dependent or independent variables. Dependent variables are dependent on the independent variables. For example, several researchers wish to determine how high-density lipoprotein (HDL) cholesterol may influence the risk of an individual for developing IHD (ischemic heart disease). The level of HDL cholesterol is the independent variable. The observed result of the development of IHD is the dependent variable, since HDL cholesterol is causally associated with the development of IHD. In this context, an independent variable is also referred to as an "explanatory variable" or a "predictor variable"; a dependent variable is also known as a "response variable" or an "outcome variable" [1].

A variable takes a number or a quantity as its value. If a person weights 76 kg, the value of the variable weight is 76 kg.

A survey or experiment yields a set of data ranging from a few measurements to thousands of observations. Table 1.1 shows aggregated data of hand, foot, and mouth disease (HFMD) cases in Beijing from September 1, 2010, to September 7, 2010. During that 1-week period of time, there were 563 HFMD cases reported to the China CDC through the National Disease Reporting Information System (NDRS).

Tables, graphs, and numerical summary measures can all be used to present data; the table above is a summary of descriptive statistics. However, the type of data must first be determined prior to the presentation of the data. The types of data are usually defined as either quantitative or qualitative data.

Quantitative variables take numerical values that arithmetic operations can be applied to; they are further divided into two types: continuous and discrete variables. The following table (Table 1.2) presents the individual records for the HFMD cases from the data in Table 1.1. In Table 1.2, age is a continuous variable, since it takes numeric values and arithmetic operations can be applied to it. For example, the average age and difference of them between the two groups could be calculated from the data. A discrete variable only takes integers, such as the number of patients in a hospital in January, the number of newborns in a county, the number of injuries that a person sustained in the last 3 months, etc.

Qualitative data also consist of two types of variables: categorical and ordinal variables. Categorical variables describe the data in terms of some quality or categorization, including well-defined aspects of the variable (e.g., gender, nationality, ethnicity, yes or no, life or death, pass or fail). Severity, another type of qualitative variable, is denoted as mild, moderate, or severe in the following table. It is known as an ordinal variable, since serious order of mild, moderate, and severe cases exists.

Table 1.1 Reported HFMD cases during a 1-week period in Beijing

Areas	Cases	Deaths	With severity
District	542	2	12
County	21	3	12
Total	563	5	24

Table 1.2 Individual HFMD cases reported to the China CDC during a 1-week period in Beijing

ID	Age (years)	Gender	Severity	Lab-confirmed
1	5	Female	Mild	No
2	3	Female	Mild	No
3	1	Male	Moderate	No
...	...	...	...	...
562	7	Male	Severe	Yes
563	9	Female	Mild	No

1.3 Probabilities

The results of surveys or experiments are events or basic elements to which probability can be applied. Outcomes such as lung cancer, whether a student passes an examination, or whether a 40-year-old man lives in the next 5 years, are all considered events. Uppercase, or capital, letters usually represent such events. There are several operations that can be performed on the event.

The intersection of two events A and B, denoted by A ∩ B, is defined as the event 'both A and B' (as shown in Fig. 1.1a). Let A represent the event that a man has a stomach cancer; let B represent the event that the same man's wife suffers from a stomach cancer as well. The intersection of events A and B would be the event that both the man and his wife sustain stomach cancers.

The union of two events, A and B, is denoted by A ∪ B and defined as the event 'either A or B' or 'both A and B' (as shown in Fig. 1.1b). In the example mentioned above, the union of events A and B would be the event that either the man or his wife has a stomach cancer or that they both have stomach cancers.

The complement of an event, A, is denoted by A′ (as shown in Fig. 1.1c). The complement is the event that is "not A." Event A indicates that the man has the disease, so the complement of event A, denoted as $\bar{A}$, indicates that the man does not have the disease.

After numerous repeated trials under virtually identical conditions, the probability of an event A is the relative frequency of the occurrence according to the frequentist definition. If an experiment is repeated n times under essentially identical conditions, and if an event A occurs m times, then as n grows larger, the ratio of m to n approaches a fixed limit referred to as the probability of event A: $P(A) = \dfrac{m}{n}$.

The probability of an event takes a numerical value that lies between 0 and 1. A value of 1 indicates that a particular event occurs in each of the n trials and that the probability is $n/n = 1$. If an event can never happen, it has a probability of $0/n = 0$. As a rule of thumb, when the probability of an event occurring is less than 0.05, we tend to take it for granted that this event will not happen in a random sampling.

From the description above, we should notice that probability is a theoretical number, we cannot observe it directly in the real world, and what we can count and calculate is frequency.

Fig. 1.1 Venn diagrams showing the operations of the events

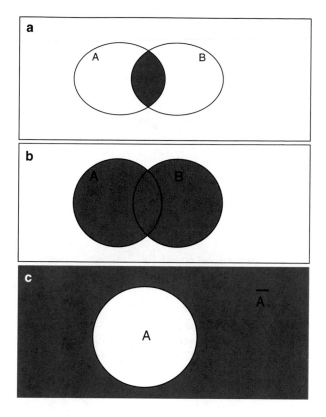

1.4 Populations and Samples

The main use of medical statistics is to infer information about the population from samples taken from that population. The population is a collection of basic elements which have the same properties according to the purpose of the study. It can include similar people, observations, or measurements, in which certain subjects can be random selected to be a sample. We often infer a property or attribute of the population by the sample taken from it. For instance, Chinese adults living in China, 12-year-old students in Beijing, or patients with diabetes mellitus in Shanghai all are populations; we can select some of them to form a random sample and then use proper statistical inference methods introduced in the following chapters with the sample at hand to draw the conclusions on the targeted population.

Sometimes, the number of subjects or individuals in a population might be too large, so a sample of that population is selected. The purpose of sampling is to select and study a part of the population to infer information for the whole population. A sampling survey of 2‰ of the population across China was conducted in 2006 in order to get an idea of the prevalence and distribution of visual, hearing, speech, physical, intellectual, and mental disabilities among Chinese people.

The values or numbers calculated from the population are often called parameters, and those derived from the sample are referred to statistics. Parameters are notated by Greek letters, such as μ, σ, ρ, etc. Statistics are represented by Latin letters, such as $\bar{x}$, s, and r, which correspond to the parameters above.

1.5   Steps of Statistical Work

The entire process of statistical work contains four steps: statistical design, data collection, data management, and data analysis. All these steps are important, and none can be ignored.

Statistical design is the first step of statistical work and is also a key step in medical research. It guides the data collection and data analysis on the right track. In this stage, the study must be carefully devised and arranged in terms of the principles of the study design, especially for sampling methods, sample size calculation, way of data collection, quality control, statistical method, as well as organization and implementation of the plan.

Data collection is the basis of statistical work. Its purpose is to collect reliable original data based on the statistical design. Data can be characterized as routine data or one-time collected data. The criteria of data are required for accuracy, completeness, timeliness, comparability, and usability.

Data management involves checking, correcting, and manipulating data to eventually make the data systematic, logical, and usable for analyses.

Data analysis, the last step of statistical work, involves statistical descriptions and inferences. A descriptive statistics describes the properties and distributions of the data using summary measurements, such as mean, standard deviation, frequency, and percentiles. A statistical inference involves inferring some attributes of the population using the information from samples under a certain confidence level or probability.

Chapter Summary
In this chapter, quantitative and qualitative data, variables, types of variables, and probability are explained and discussed. Understanding these basic concepts of medical statistics is fundamental to learn statistical description and statistical inferences.

Chapter 2
Study Design, Sample Size Estimation, and Selection of Statistical Method

Xinghua Yang and Junhui Zhang

Objectives
Study design is the first step in medical research; a well-designed study makes the research valid and reliable. In this chapter, we will introduce the common study designs in medical research—observational and experimental studies (includes laboratory studies and clinical trials). The study design includes both professional and statistical designs. In addition, we will introduce the estimation of sample size (that is an important part of the study design) and the selection of statistical methods.

Key Concepts
Study design; Sample size; Statistical principles

2.1 Introduction

The study design is the first step in medical research. A well-designed study makes the research both valid and reliable. The procedure of medical statistics begins at the study's design, including statistical design, data collection, data management, and data analysis. Study design is an important link in statistical work in medical research. A well-designed study helps get more work done in less time. Without a

X. Yang (✉)
School of Public Health, Capital Medical University, Beijing, China

J. Zhang
School of Public Health, Southwest Medical University, Luzhou, China

© Zhengzhou University Press 2024
X. Guo, F. Xue (eds.), *Textbook of Medical Statistics*,
https://doi.org/10.1007/978-981-99-7390-3_2

proper design, it is difficult to obtain both accurate data and results. Therefore, study design is an important component of medical statistics.

The design of a medical research includes statistical and professional design. Statistical design refers to the study of the problems and goals, formulation of a research plan (includes sampling plans), research project design, and sample size estimation. Professional design originates from professional knowledge, which is included in the study proposal. Statistical design is the main content of this chapter. Before researchers conduct a study, they need to consider which type of study design to apply, determine how to collect the data, design a sampling plan, estimate the size of the sample, select a suitable analysis method, and write a corresponding research plan. Only afterward can they draw a reliable conclusion. A well-designed research study obtains reliable results using lower costs of manpower, less time and money, higher efficiency, and ability to estimate the random error within the observed data.

According to the research target, study design, and statistical analysis plan, the data can be analyzed using the appropriate statistical methods after it has been collected and sorted.

2.2 Design of Observational Studies

Observational study designs are common in medical studies, such as cross-sectional studies, case-control studies, and cohort studies.

Cross-sectional studies form a class of research methods that involve all of the observations of a population at a defined time, and their aim is to provide data on the entire population of the study, whereas case-control studies typically include only the sample of individuals with a specific disease. They can also be used to describe a certain feature of the population, such as the prevalence of an illness, or to support inferences of a causal relationship. Cohort studies differ from both by making a series of observations on members of the studied population over a period of time.

2.2.1 Cross-Sectional Study

Cross-sectional studies involve data collected at a defined time. They are often used to assess the prevalence of acute or chronic conditions or to determine the results of a medical intervention. They may take the form of a census or sampling survey.

The goals of cross-sectional studies are (1) to find out how widely an existing disease prevails in different geographical areas, among different populations, and at different times, as well as what factors the disease is associated with, in order to determine who is at risk of contracting the disease, and (2) to detect patients for early treatment and prevent the disease from progressing.

For example, we want to measure BMI in a population. We could randomly draw a sample of 2000 people from the population (supposed there are 200,000 people in the population), measure their weight and height, and calculate what percentage of that sample is categorized as obese. For example, 30% of our sample was categorized as obese. Please note the cross-sectional sample provides us with a snapshot of that population at that one point in time; we do not know if obesity is increasing or decreasing based on one cross-sectional sample; we can only describe the current situation.

The advantages of a cross-sectional study are that it is easily carried out, can observe many diseases and risk factors in the same time, save much labor, resources, and time, etc.

The biases of this study are nonresponse, recall bias or report bias, and measuring bias.

Usually, there are four random sampling methods used to draw a random sample from a population.

1. Simple random sampling: Simple random sampling is probably the most intuitive form of random sampling and suitable for small populations, since every individual has the same probability of being sampled. For example, suppose 100 college students want to get a ticket for a football game, but there are only 10 tickets for them, so they decide to have a fair way to see who goes. So everyone is given a number in the range from 0 to 99, and random numbers are generated, either electronically or from a table of random numbers. Numbers outside the range from 0 to 99 are ignored. The first ten numbers would identify the lucky ticket winners. Simple random sampling is the simplest of the probability sampling techniques. It requires a complete sampling frame, which may not be available or feasible to construct for large populations. Even if a complete frame is available, more efficient approaches may be possible if other useful information is available about the units in the population.

2. Systematic sampling: Systematic sample is useful when the population has a sequence (such as an ID code), and according to the sequence of the individuals, subjects are sampled at a fixed interval. With systematic random sampling, we create a list of every member of the population. From the list, we randomly select the first sample element from the first k elements on the population list. Thereafter, we select every kth element on the list. For instance, suppose we want to draw 10 rooms from 100 rooms in a building. $100/10 = 10$, so every 10th room is chosen after a random starting point between 1 and 10 (using simple random sampling). If the random starting point is 6, then the rooms selected are 6, 16, 26, etc.; 86; and 96. As an aside, if every tenth room was a "north facing room," then this could destroy the randomness of the sample. Systematic sampling is different from simple random sampling, since every possible sample of n elements is not equally likely. It is to be applied only if the given population is logically homogeneous, because systematic sample units are uniformly distributed over the population. The researcher must ensure that the chosen sampling interval does not hide a pattern. Any pattern would threaten randomness.

3. Stratified sampling: Stratified sampling controls for confounding factors that may influence the results of the study when a population is stratified. Therefore, the individuals in each stratum are randomly sampled. With stratified sampling, the population is divided into groups based on some characteristic. Then, within each group, a probability sample (often a simple random sample) is selected. In stratified sampling, the groups are called strata. As an example, suppose we conduct a national survey. We might divide the population into groups or strata, based on geography—North, South, East, and West. Then, within each stratum, we might randomly select survey respondents.

4. Cluster sampling: If the individuals belong to a certain unit (such as a community, school, class, city, county), then the entire unit may be directly sampled, instead of the individuals. With cluster sampling, every member of the population is assigned to one, and only one group. Each group is called a cluster. A sample of clusters is chosen, using a probability method (often simple random sampling). Only individuals within sampled clusters are surveyed. Note the difference between cluster sampling and stratified sampling. With stratified sampling, the sample includes elements from each stratum. With cluster sampling, in contrast, the sample includes elements only from sampled clusters.

Among these four types of sampling methods, the sampling error from the largest to the smallest is cluster sampling > simple random sampling > systematic sampling > stratified sampling.

2.2.2   Case-Control Study

A case-control study is a type of epidemiological study design. It is typically used for retrospective studies but can also be applied to prospective studies. In a case-control study, subjects that have a disease are chosen as cases and those without the disease as controls. Data on those individuals are collected, and comparisons are made between cases and controls to determine whether any characteristics differ between the two groups.

There are two types of case-control study, matched case-control study and group case-control study. Matched case-control studies have two types—frequency matching case-control studies and individual matching case-control studies. A frequently matched case-control study matches the control group with the disease group by the proportion of exposed characteristics. An individual matching case-control study matches the control group by individuals, and the analysis based on such matched sets promotes statistical power. When one case matches one control only, it is called a 1:1 matched design or paired design. When one case matches two controls, it is called a 1:2 matched design.

In case-control studies, data are not available to calculate the incidence rate of the disease being studied, and the actual relative risk cannot be determined. The measure of association between exposure and occurrence of disease in case-control studies is the so-called odds ratio (the ratio of odds of exposure in diseased subjects

Table 2.1 Case-control study design

Exposure	Disease	
	Yes (cases)	No (controls)
Yes	a	b
No	c	d
Odds of exposure	a/c	b/d

to the odds of exposure in the non-diseased). The following Table 2.1 exemplifies the basic method of calculating the odds ratio in a case-control study.

The odds ratio (OR): Odds is the ratio of exposured and non-exposured number of people in the case or control group; then the odds of case group divided the odds of control group; we call the quotient is odds ratio. That is, ratio of odds of exposure is thus given by a/c:b/d (or ad/bc). The odds ratio is generally a good estimate of the relative risk when the disease rate is low. The terms "odds ratio" and "relative risk" are in fact interchangeable when used in case-control studies.

One of the most significant case-control studies was the demonstration of the link between tobacco smoking and lung cancer by Sir Richard Doll and others after him. Doll was able to show a statistically significant association between the two in a large case-control study.

This kind of study tends to be less costly to carry out than prospective cohort studies, as well as having the potential to be shorter in duration. Another aspect is the greater statistical power of this type of study in several situations, given the fact that cohort studies must often wait for a "sufficient" number of disease events to be accrued.

Such studies have pointed the way to a number of important discoveries and advances, but their retrospective, non-randomized nature limits the strength of their conclusions. Case-control studies are a relatively inexpensive and frequently used type of epidemiological study that can be carried out by small teams.

Case-control studies are observational in nature and thus do not provide the same level of evidence as randomized controlled trials. The results may be confounded by other factors, to the extent of giving the opposite answer to better studies. It may also be more difficult to establish the timeline of exposure to disease outcome in the setting of a case-control study than within a prospective cohort study design where the exposure is ascertained prior to following the subjects over time in order to ascertain their outcome status.

The other most important drawback in case-control studies relates to the difficulty of obtaining reliable information about an individual's exposure status over time. But many high quality and reliable case-control studies have been carried out and have produced useful results.

2.2.3   Cohort Study

A cohort study is also called a prospective study, follow-up study, or panel study. It is a form of longitudinal study used in medicine and social science. Crucially, the cohort is identified before the appearance of the disease under investigation. The study groups follow a group of people who do not have the disease for a period of time and see who develops the disease (new incidence). The cohort cannot therefore be defined as a group of people who already have the disease. Prospective (longitudinal) cohort studies examining the link between exposure and disease strongly aid in studying causal associations, though distinguishing true causality usually requires further corroboration from additional experimental trials. A cohort is a group of people who share a common characteristic or experience within a defined period (e.g., exposure to a drug or vaccine). The comparison group may be the general population from which the cohort is drawn, or it may be another cohort of persons thought to have had little or no exposure to the substance under investigation, but otherwise similar. Alternatively, subgroups within the cohort may be compared to each other.

The starting point of a cohort study is the recording of healthy subjects with and without exposure to the putative agent or the characteristic being studied. Individuals exposed to the agent under study are followed over time, and their health status is observed and recorded during the course of the study. In order to compare the occurrence of disease in exposed subjects to its occurrence in nonexposed subjects, the health status of a group of individuals not exposed to the agent under study is also followed.

The measure of disease in cohort studies is the incidence rate, which is the proportion of subjects who develop the disease under study within a specified time period. We use the person-years of observation to calculate the incidence rates for exposed and nonexposed subjects separately.

The measure of association between exposure and disease in cohort studies is the relative risk. The relative risk is the ratio of the incidence rate of index subjects to that of control subjects. A relative risk of 1.0 signifies that the incidence rate is the same among exposed and nonexposed subjects, indicating a lack of association between exposure and disease. A relative risk of less than 1.0 provides evidence for a protective effect of exposure, whereas a relative risk above 1.0 suggests that exposed people are at a higher risk than nonexposed persons.

The advantage of prospective cohort study data is that it can help determine risk factors for contracting a new disease, because it is a longitudinal observation of the individual through time, and the collection of data at regular intervals, so recall error is reduced. However, cohort studies are expensive to conduct, are sensitive to attrition, and take a long follow-up time to generate useful data. Prospective cohort studies are considered to yield the most reliable results in observational epidemiology. They enable a wide range of exposure-disease associations to be studied.

2.3 Design of Experimental Studies

In general usage, experimental design is the design of any information-gathering exercises where variation is present, whether under the full control of the experimenter or not. In the design of experiments, the experimenter is often interested in the effect of interventions (treatments) on subjects. Design of experiments is thus a discipline that has very broad application across all the natural and social sciences.

2.3.1 *Statistical Principles of Experimental Study Design*

In experimental studies, three statistical principles during the design stage of an experiment must be followed in order to control for the random error, avoid, or reduce the nonrandom errors, in which they are randomization, control, and replication.

2.3.1.1 Randomization

In the design of experiments, randomization involves randomly allocating the experimental units across the treatment groups. For example, if an experiment compares a new drug against a standard drug, then the patients should be allocated to either the new drug or to the standard drug control using randomization.

Randomization enhances the consistency of distributions of many uncontrolled nontreatment factors among the compared groups. Randomization should be carried out during the process of sampling and allocation. In random sampling, each subject who meets the experimental condition has the same opportunity to be selected. In other words, each individual within the population has the same probability of being in the sample. As to random allocation, each subject has the same probability of being assigned to each of the experiment groups. Here, random sampling guarantees a representative sample, and the conclusion can be generalized to the population; random grouping enhances the balance and comparability among compared groups.

2.3.1.2 Control

A study is always based on a rational comparison. A proper control group must be established in order to manifest the effect of the treatment. The balance between the control and treatment groups is the premise that ensures the correct manifestation of experimental effects. Balance refers to the fact that among the compared groups, only the treatment factors are different, and the distribution of those important, controllable nontreatment factors should be kept consistent for as long as possible. For example, the characteristics of the experimental subjects within different contrast groups should be kept consistent on the distributions of gender, age, and health conditions. In medical research, the constitution of the control group must meet the following three conditions:

(a) Homogeneity: Except for treatment factors, the control group must have the same nontreatment factors as the treatment groups do.
(b) Synchronization: Once the control and treatment groups are established, the entire research process for both groups must take place in the same time and space.
(c) Specificity: The control group should be established exclusively for the relevant treatment groups being studied.

After establishing the control group, the baseline conditions of all of the compared groups should be examined for balance. There are several types of control groups: empty control (placebo control), experimental control, mutual control, self-control, standard control, and historical control.

2.3.1.3 Replication

Replication involves taking a number of observations under the same experimental condition so as to improve the reliability and validity of experimental results. Replication implies (1) replication of the whole experiment; (2) carrying out the experiment with several experimental units; and (3) repeated observations on the same experimental unit.

Replication makes the experiment replicable and improves its reliability. It also avoids applying specific results to universal populations or viewing coincidences as influencing factors. Thus, replication aims to enhance the precision of a measurement.

From the probability theory, the more an experiment is repeated, the closer the parameter and sample statistic (i.e., sample frequency, sample mean, etc.). However, repeating an experiment too many times and making too many observations wastes resources. Researchers may also fail to control the experimental condition efficiently, which lowers the reliability of the experimental results. One purpose of statistical design is to estimate an adequate sample size to make a reliable statistical conclusion and avoid unnecessary waste.

2.3.2 Basic Elements of Experimental Study Design

In addition to above three statistical principles, there are three elements that should be considered: treatment, subject, and effect. For example, to evaluate the effect of a hypoglycemic drug in an experiment, the treatment is use or nonuse of the hypoglycemic drug, the subjects are diabetic patients, and the effect is the amount of blood sugar.

2.3.2.1 Treatment

Treatment factors generally refer to externally applied factors (such as a drug, a type of surgery, etc.), and sometimes the subject's own characteristics such as gender, age, occupation, educational level, ethnicity, marital status, etc. Treatment factors can be divided into single and multiple factors.

1. **Grasp the main factors in the experiment.** The main factors of a trial should be determined as treatment factors according to the purpose of the study. Treatment factors of a trial should not be too much. You should choose several major or key factors as treatment factors.

2. **Identify treatment factors and confounding factors**. Confounding factors are the factors that affect the experimental effects and coexist with the treatment factors. They usually distribute unevenly between experimental and control groups, resulting in a distorted relationship between treatment and experimental effects. Confounding factors might have a confounding effect on the results of the study. Therefore, we should seek to eliminate the interference from confounding factors. The main method to eliminate confounding effect is to balance the experimental treatment group and the control group.

3. **Standardize treatment factors**. Treatment factors should be unchanged throughout the experiment, since changes in treatment factors will affect the evaluation of test results.

2.3.2.2 Subject

A subject is someone or something that undergoes testing in a scientific experiment. The choice of subjects is the key to successful experiment.

1. **Human subject.** Human in treatment group and control group should have similar demographic factors, such as gender, age, nationality, occupation, education level, economic status, etc.

2. **Animal subject.** Animal in intervention group and control group should have similar species, strain, age, gender, weight, nutritional status, etc.

2.3.2.3 Effect

Experimental effect is a reaction or result of a treatment factor acting on a subject, which is represented by observation indicators. Observation indicators include the selection of experimental outcome indicators and the observation of indicators.

1. **Selection of experimental outcome indicators.** Observed indicators of experimental effects should be selected with strong objectivity, high sensitivity, and good accuracy. Quantitative indicators should be selected as far as possible when designing, such as fasting blood glucose (FBG), 2 h postprandial blood glucose (2Hbg), and hemoglobin (HbA1c).

2. **Observation of indicators.** When observing the experimental effects, bias should be avoided, and blind methods should be used in designing.

2.3.3 Common Experimental Designs

2.3.3.1 Completely Randomized Design

A completely randomized design randomly allocates the homogeneous subjects into two or more groups.

Example 2.1 Randomly allocate ten female mice of similar weight into two groups (use the Appendix: random digits table).

Firstly, ten female mice are numbered from 1 to 10. Secondly, we copy 10 random numbers from left to right on 20th row and first column in the appendix "random digits table." Thirdly, we sort the random numbers from the minimum to the maximum. And define the rules in advance that the mice corresponding to the odd random numbers are assigned to the A group, and those corresponding to the even numbers are assigned to the B group. At last, we get the result of random allocation of ten mice: A group includes mice 2, 4, 6, 7, and 8, and B group includes mice 1, 3, 5, 9, and 10. The assigning process is shown in Table 2.2.

For completely randomized designs, the levels of the primary factor are randomly assigned to the experimental units. The run sequence of the experimental units is also determined randomly. In practice, randomization is typically performed by a computer program. However, randomization can also be generated from random digits tables or by some physical mechanism (e.g., drawing slips of paper).

2.3.3.2 Randomized Paired Design

One such randomized design is the randomized paired design. Two individuals similar in terms of several important features are paired, and two individuals of any pair are randomly assigned to receive two treatments. For instance, two animals of the same gender and from the same nest could be paired. Any specimen can be divided into two parts as a pair. For any individual, pretreatment and posttreatment can be regarded as a pair. The special characteristic of the data under paired design is a one-to-one correspondence, since researchers are concerned with the difference of the effects within the pair rather than the effect on each individual.

Example 2.2 Separately using two measurement instruments of blood lead to measure ten children's blood lead levels (µg/L), and obtaining the data in Table 2.3, are the results of the two methods different?

Here, the ten pairs of measurements of the children are shown that the two measures of each child are relative.

Table 2.2 Ten female mice were randomly assigned to two groups

Mice	1	2	3	4	5	6	7	8	9	10
Random number	31	16	93	32	43	50	27	89	87	19
Sorting random number	4	1	10	5	6	7	3	9	8	2
Grouping result	B	A	B	A	B	A	A	A	B	B

Table 2.3 Ten children's blood lead levels (μg/L) using two ways

ID	Method A	Method B
1	67	71
2	101	105
3	23	28
4	55	54
5	135	146
6	96	101
7	120	130
8	74	81
9	115	113
10	88	93

2.3.3.3 Randomized Block Design

Randomized block design is useful when a confounding factor contributes to the variation. Age is frequently a confounding factor in medical studies, so investigators often apply control subjects matched on age with treatment subjects.

In a randomized block design, subjects are first subdivided into homogeneous blocks based on a confounding factor or more; then subjects from each block are randomly assigned to each level of the experimental factor. This type of study is especially useful in laboratory experiments in which investigators are concerned about genetic variation and its effect on the outcome being studied. Litters of animals are defined as the blocks, and littermates are then randomly assigned to the different levels of treatment. In this experiment, blocking is used to control for genetic differences.

Example 2.3 12 white mice randomly allocated into three groups: **A**, **B**, and **C**.

Here, we plan to randomize the 12 white mice into 3 groups. Firstly, according to the nest, we assign the white mice into four blocks and then code the mice. Secondly, we copy 12 randomized numbers from left to right beginning with sixth row and first column in the appendix "table of random digit." Thirdly, sort the random numbers from the smallest to the largest in each block group (nest). And define the rules in advance that the white mice whose corresponding sorting random number in each block is 1, 2, and 3 will be assigned to A, B, and C group, respectively. At last, we get the assigning result: A group includes mice 1.1, 2.2, 3.2, and 4.2; B group includes mice 1.2, 2.3, 3.1, and 4.3; and C group includes mice 1.3, 2.1, 3.3, and 4.1. The assigning process is shown in Table 2.4.

Table 2.4 12 white mice randomly allocated into3 groups

Block	I			II			III			IV		
White mice	1.1	1.2	1.3	2.1	2.2	2.3	3.1	3.2	3.3	4.1	4.2	4.3
Random number	16	22	77	94	39	49	54	43	54	82	17	37
Sorting random number	1	2	3	3	1	2	2	1	3	3	1	2
Assigning result	A	B	C	C	A	B	B	A	C	C	A	B

2.3.4 Clinical Trials

Clinical trials are sets of tests in medical research and drug development that generate safety and efficacy data for health interventions (e.g., drugs, diagnostics, devices, therapy protocols).

Depending on the type of product and the stage of its development, investigators initially enroll healthy volunteers and/or patients into pilot studies, followed by a larger-scale study that often compares the new product with the currently prescribed treatment. As safety and efficacy data are gathered, the number of patients is typically increased. Clinical trials can vary in size from a single center in one country to multicenter trials in multiple countries.

Clinical trials may be designed to do the following:

- Assess the safety and effectiveness of a new medication or device for a specific kind of patient (e.g., patients diagnosed with Alzheimer's disease).
- Assess the safety and effectiveness of a different dose of a medication than is commonly used (e.g., 10 mg dosage instead of the usual 5 mg dosage).

Because the clinical trial is designed to test hypotheses and rigorously monitor and assess what happens, clinical trials can be seen as an application of the scientific method. More specifically, clinical trials are sometimes regarded as the experimental step to understanding human or animal biology.

Randomized controlled trials (RCT) are a superior methodology in the hierarchy of evidence in the research. They limit the potential for any biases by randomly assigning one patient pool to an intervention and another patient pool to a nonintervention (or placebo). This minimizes the chance that the incidence of confounding variables (particularly unknown confounding variables) will differ between the two groups (Fig. 2.1).

A randomized controlled trial is a type of experimental study where subjects are randomly assigned to either a control or intervention group, where something is done to the intervention group (they are given drugs, educational seminars, counseling, etc.), and then scientists see if the outcomes are different between the two groups.

When trying to determine whether a drug or intervention is effective at treating or preventing a disease, a randomized controlled trial is often considered to be the gold standard. This is due to the fact that it is easier to get a good idea of causation with a randomized trial, as opposed to an observational study. The only thing different between the two groups is whether they received the drug; if the subjects who

Fig. 2.1 Population hierarchy for an intervention study

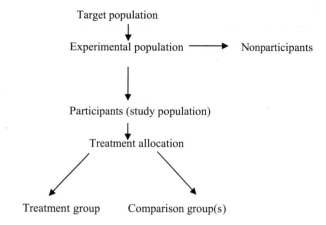

received the drug had better outcomes, there is a reasonable chance that the drug caused the outcome. In other types of studies, subtle but important differences are harder to control.

There are two processes involved in randomizing patients to different interventions. First is choosing a randomization procedure to generate an unpredictable sequence of allocations. The second and more practical issue is allocation concealment, which refers to the stringent precautions taken to ensure that the group assignment of patients is not revealed prior to definitively allocating them to their respective groups. A blind experiment is a scientific experiment where some of the persons involved are prevented from knowing certain information that might lead to conscious or unconscious bias on their part, which could invalidate the results.

2.3.5   Quasi-Experiments

The design of a quasi-experiment relates to the setting up a particular type of an experiment or study in which one has little or no control over the allocation of the treatments or other factors being studied. The key difference in this empirical approach is the lack of random assignment. Experiments designed in this manner are referred to as having a quasi-experimental design, for example, interrupted time series designs (ITS), before-after study, regression discontinuity design, etc.

2.4   Sample Size

Researchers must learn how large a sample is needed when beginning their research, because they may not be able to determine the significance when it occurs. When considering the sample size, we usually care both type I and type II errors for two common situations: a study that involves one or two means and one or two proportions.

In addition to previously mentioned conditions, the determination of sample size involves many other factors. For instance, the sample size for a quantitative index is less than that for a qualitative index. Under the same test level and test power, the sample size of a one-sided test is less than that of a two-sided test.

2.4.1 Experimental Sample Size: Proportion

2.4.1.1 Sample Size for Studies with One Proportion

The researcher must answer four questions prior to estimating the sample size needed for a single proportion: (1) What is the desired level of significance (the α level) related to the null hypothesis, π_0? (2) What level of power $(1 - \beta)$ is desired to associate with the alternative hypothesis, π_1? (3) How large should the difference be between the proportions $(\pi_1 - \pi_0)$ for it to be clinically significant? (4) What is a good estimate of the standard deviation in the population?

Specifications of α for a null hypothesis and β for an alternative hypothesis permit us to solve for the sample size. These specifications lead to the following two critical ratios, where Z_a is the two-tailed value (for a two-sided test) of Z related to α (generally 0.05) and Z_β is the lower one-tailed value of Z related to β (generally 0.20). We use the lower one-sided value for β, because we want the power to be equal to $(1 - \beta)$ or more.

For a proportion, it is easy to determine the estimated standard deviation of the proportion π, which is $\pi(1 - \pi)$.

The formula to determine the sample size is:

$$n = \left(\frac{Z_{\alpha/2} + Z_\beta}{\delta}\right)^2 \pi\left(1 - \pi\right). \tag{2.1}$$

where $Z_{a/2}$ is the two-tailed Z value related to the null hypothesis and Z_β is the lower one-tailed Z value related to the alternative hypothesis.

Example 2.4 A doctor uses Chinese traditional medicine to treat the patients with chronic pelvic inflammatory disease, and the observed relapse rate is 16%. The known relapse rate using Western medicine is 46%. Given $\alpha = 0.05$ and $\beta = 0.10$, how many people are needed to carry out this clinical trial?

According to the aim of this example, $\pi = 0.46$, $\delta = 0.46–0.16 = 0.30$, $Z_{a/2} = 1.96$, and $Z_\beta = 1.282$:

$$n = \left(\frac{Z_{\alpha/2} + Z_\beta}{\delta}\right)^2 \pi\left(1 - \pi\right) = \left(\frac{1.96 + 1.282}{0.30}\right)^2 \times 0.45 \times \left(1 - 0.45\right) = 28.9$$

Twenty-nine patients are expected to be required in this clinical trial.

2.4.1.2   Sample Size for Studies with Two Proportions

The formula to determine the sample size is:

$$n_1 = n_2 = \frac{2\left(Z_{\alpha/2} + Z_\beta\right)^2 \pi\left(1-\pi\right)}{\delta^2}. \tag{2.2}$$

where $Z_{\alpha/2}$ is the two-tailed Z value related to the null hypothesis and Z_β is the lower one-tailed Z value related to the alternative hypothesis. $\pi = (\pi_1 + \pi_2)/2$, where π_1 and π_2 are the population proportions of the comparative groups.

Example 2.5 After studying whether the hookworm infectious rate is different between vegetable farmers and grain farmers, we know that the infectious rate of vegetable farmers and grain farmers is 20% and 10%, respectively. Given $\alpha = 0.05$ and $\beta = 0.10$, how many people are needed to be surveyed when the two group numbers are equal?

The efficacies of drugs A and B in the treatment of eczema were observed. The effective rates of drugs A and B were 60% and 86%, respectively. Given $\alpha = 0.05$ and $\beta = 0.10$, how many people are needed to carry out this clinical trial when the two group numbers are equal?

According to the example, $\pi_1 = 60\%$, $\pi_2 = 86\%$, $\pi = 0.73$, $\delta = 0.26$, $Z_{\alpha/2} = 1.96$, and $Z_\beta = 1.282$:

$$n_1 = n_2 = \frac{2\left(Z_{\alpha/2} + Z_\beta\right)^2 \pi\left(1-\pi\right)}{\delta^2} = \frac{2 \times (1.96 + 1.282)^2 \times 0.73 \times (1 - 0.73)}{0.26^2} = 61.3$$

The sample size in each group is 62.

2.4.2   Experimental Sample Size: Mean

2.4.2.1   Sample Size for Studies with One Mean

Similar to estimating the sample size for a single proportion, researchers must also answer four questions to estimate the sample size needed for a single mean: (1) What level of significance (α level) related to the null hypothesis is wanted? (2) What is the desired level of power (equal to $1 - \beta$)? (3) How large should the difference be between the mean and the standard value or norm ($\mu_1 - \mu_0$) in order to be clinically important? (4) What is the estimate of the standard deviation of σ?

$$n = \left[\frac{\left(Z_{\alpha/2} + Z_\beta\right)\sigma}{\delta}\right]^2. \tag{2.3}$$

The symbols in the formula are the same as before; σ is the population standard deviation, which can be replaced by sample standard deviation.

2.4.2.2 Sample Size for Studies with Two Means

The formula to determine the sample size is:

$$n_1 = n_2 = 2\left[\frac{\left(Z_{\alpha/2} + Z_\beta\right)\sigma}{\delta}\right]^2.$$ (2.4)

where n_1 and n_2 are the sample sizes.

Example 2.6 Comparing the effectiveness of Drug A and Drug B for improving anemia from prior experience, on the average, Drug A increases hemoglobin 1.5 g/L and Drug B increases hemoglobin 2.5 g/L, if σ = 1.7 g/L. Given α = 0.05 and β = 0.20, how many Q group if each group number is equal?

Our example, σ = 1.7 g/L, δ = (2.5–1.5) = 1.0 g/L, $Z_{\alpha/2}$ = 1.96, Z_β = 0.842

$$n_1 = n_2 = 2\left[\frac{\left(Z_{\alpha/2} + Z_\beta\right)\sigma}{\delta}\right]^2 = 2 \times \left[\frac{(1.96 + 0.842) \times 1.7}{1}\right]^2 = 45.4$$

The sample size in each group is equal to 46, for a total of 92 cases.

2.4.3 Estimation of Sample Size for a Case-Control Study

Several formulas can be used to estimate the sample size for a case-control study. Estimation is completed in two steps. The first step is to calculate N by using the formula:

$$N' = \frac{\left[Z_\alpha \sqrt{(1 + 1/C)PQ} + Z_\beta \sqrt{P_1 Q_1 + P_0 Q_0 / C}\right]^2}{\left(P_1 - P_0\right)^2}.$$ (2.5)

where C = ratio of the number of controls to the number of cases given in advance. For example, if equal sample sizes in both case and control groups are planned, then C = 1.0. P_0 is the estimated proportion of individuals exposed to the risk factor in the control population. $Q_0 = 1 - P_0$ is the proportion of individuals without exposure in the control population.

$$P_1 = \frac{P_0 RR}{\left[1 + P_0 (RR - 1)\right]}.$$ (2.6)

P_1 is the estimated proportion of cases exposed to the risk factor in the case population. $Q_1 = 1 - P_1$ is the proportion of cases without exposure in the case population. RR is the estimate of relative risk under the alternative hypothesis, and

$$P = \frac{P_1 + P_0}{2}, Q = (1 - P). \tag{2.7}$$

Z_a is the standard normal deviation with the probability of type I error α, and $\alpha = 0.05$ is usually used. Thus, the one-sided value is $Z_{0.05} = 1.645$, and the two-sided value is $Z_{0.05} = 1.96$.

Z_β is the standard normal deviation with the probability of type II error β. $\beta = 0.10$ is usually used, thus one-sided value $Z_{0.1} = 1.282$.

The second step is to calculate the sample size N for the case group. The formula is:

$$N = \left(\frac{N'}{4}\right)\left(1 + \sqrt{1 + \frac{4}{N'\delta}}\right)^2. \tag{2.8}$$

where $\delta = |P_1 - P_0|$.

2.5   Selection of Statistical Methods

2.5.1   The Basic Rules of Selecting Statistical Methods

In practical work, how to choose the appropriate statistical methods to analyze data is the most important and difficult question. This section shows the basic flow when choosing a statistical method according to the research purpose, design type, and data type to consider.

2.5.1.1   If There Is a Clear Research Purpose, There Would Be a Clear Analysis Goal

The research purpose is the first question to consider when selecting an appropriate statistical method. If the purpose is not clear, then data analyses would be wrong and meaningless. For example, there is no difference, we can undertake the statistical analysis at least as follows: difference Chi-square test, independence chi-square test, coefficient of association, kappa coefficient, *OR* value, *RR* value, sensitivity, specificity, etc. The index being calculated and statistical methods used for the analysis depends on the research purpose and the corresponding study design.

2.5.1.2   Select a Statistical Method According to the Type of the Study Design

The study design is another important factor in selecting statistical methods. From the experimental study design perspective, the most common design type is a completely randomized design, and the second is a paired or randomized block design.

The observational study design usually equates to the completely randomized design from the statistical point of view. Therefore, the data analysis of an observational study design and completely random design may apply a two-sample t-test, one-way analysis of variance, chi-square test, and rank sum test. For the data analysis of a paired or randomized block design, one can use a paired t-test, two-way analysis of variance, paired chi-square test, Wilcoxon's signed rank test, and Kruskal-Wallis test.

2.5.1.3   Select a Statistical Method According to the Type of Data

Data type is the third important factor in choosing a statistical method. Continuous variables correspond to the statistical method as follows: t-test, analysis of variance, correlation, and simple linear regression; categorical variables usually correspond to the statistical methods such as the chi-square test; and ordinal variables generally use the rank sum test.

The following flow chart about choosing the appropriate statistical method is shown in Fig. 2.2.

2.5.2   Case Analysis

We planned to explore the relationship between BMI and blood sugar level. We collected data for 477 patients in the checkup in the hospital (Example 2.7). How to manage and analyze these data? At first, we need to clean the data; at this step, we found that 14 patients' data were missed; and second, we plan to analyze part of data (30%) according to the statistical aim. What statistical method should be selected when we analyze data?

Example 2.7   When cleaning the medical data of 477 patients, the records that missed the important variable were deleted. In total, 463 cases were kept. To facilitate the analysis, 30% of the subjects were sampled in those 463 cases, in order to get 153 cases (see data file named Example 2.7). The main analysis variables are age, gender, height, weight, body mass index, fasting blood sugar, and grade of body mass index. BMI classification: Less than 18.5 = underweight; 18.5–24 = normal; 24–27 = overweight; and 27 and above = obese. The researchers plan to explore whether the height, weight, and grades of BMI differ between genders, what the relationship between height and weight is, and what the relationship between fasting blood sugar level and obesity grades is? Try to analyze the data.

Solution

Firstly, we do a descriptive analysis: check the frequency table, use the quantitative index to do a normal test, and calculate the averages, median, standard deviation, and quartile range. Categorical variables will be counted by categories. The

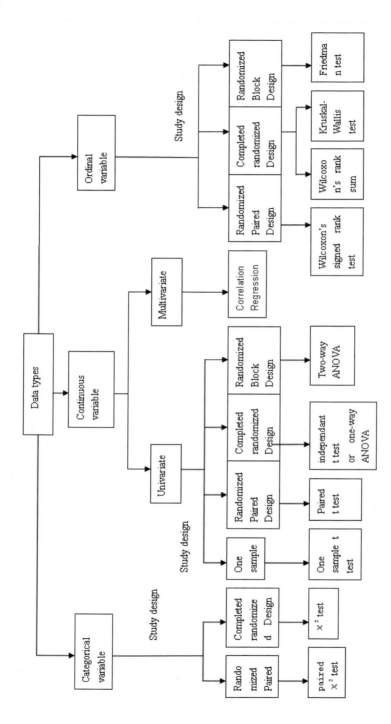

Fig. 2.2 Flow chart of appropriately choosing a statistical analysis method

Table 2.5 Main study designs in the medical research

Method	Main types
Observational study designs	Cross-sectional study Case-control study Cohort study
Experimental study designs	Randomized paired design Completely randomized design Randomized block design
Quasi-experiment designs	Randomized controlled trials ITS, before-after study Regression discontinuity design, etc.

second step is to write a statistical analysis plan (SAP) according to the research objective.

Based on the research purpose, researchers worked out the following statistical analysis plans:

1. Descriptive analysis of variables: Conduct a normal test, and calculate the mean and standard deviation of the continuous variable.
2. Compare the differences of the height and weight between genders.
3. Compare the difference of the grades of BMI between genders.
4. Analyze the relationship between height and weight.
5. Analyze the relationship between fasting blood sugar level and obesity grades.

Chapter Summary

1. The study design is the first step of conducting a medical research; a well-designed study makes the research valid and reliable. The procedure for medical statistics work includes statistical design, data collection, data management, and data analysis (four stages in total). The study design is an important bridge linking to statistical work in medical research.

   The main study designs are as follows (Table 2.5):

2. Researchers must learn how large a sample is needed before beginning their research to determine the significance when it occurs. There are several formulas that protect against both type I and type II errors for two common situations: studies that involve either one mean or one proportion and studies that measure a group twice and compare the differences before and after an intervention.
3. In practical work, knowing how to choose the appropriate statistical methods to analyze data is the most important and most difficult question. The basic ideas and principles considered in correctly choosing statistical methods are the research purpose, the type of study design, and the type of data.

Chapter 3
Statistical Tables and Graphs

Zhihang Peng and Yuxue Bi

Objectives

Statistical tables and graphs are important and useful means of summarizing and displaying numerical data. The objective of this chapter is to introduce rules and demands of making statistical tables and graphs, to learn various charts fitting to different types of data, and to make all kinds of statistical tables and graphs using the SPSS software.

Key Concepts

Statistical tables; Graphs/charts/plots; Bar charts; Histograms; Stem-and-leaf plot; Pie charts; Line charts; Scatter plots; Box plots; Mean and standard error chart

3.1 Introduction

Statistical tables and graphs are widely used to describe and summarize a set of data in medical statistics. The summarized data in tables and graphs allow us to visualize the distribution and gain useful information from the data.

Z. Peng (✉)
School of Public Health, Nanjing Medical University, Nanjing, China

Y. Bi
School of Public Health, Xi'an Jiaotong University, Xi'an, China

© Zhengzhou University Press 2024
X. Guo, F. Xue (eds.), *Textbook of Medical Statistics*,
https://doi.org/10.1007/978-981-99-7390-3_3

3.2   Structures and Types of Tables

A table is a simple method to summarize a set of observations, usually for different types of numerical data. Table 3.1 is an example of tables, which includes only one grouping variable (treatment). This simple table is also known as a one-dimension table. Tables can also include more than one grouping variable (e.g., grouping data based on treatment and county) to form a combinative table, as shown in Table 3.2.

3.3   Basic Rules and Demands for Tables

Statistical tables are most informative when they are not overly complex. As a general rule, tables should always be clearly labeled. If units of measurement are involved, they should be specified.

The title should briefly describe the content of the table, which includes the time and place of the observations and always label a serial number that is located at the top of the table.

Headings of statistical tables include row and column headings that show the subjects and predicates of the observations, respectively. Headings should be simple and clear.

The lines of a statistical table should be as less as possible, usually a three-line table recommended—the cap line, the bottom line, and the line between the column heading and the observations. In order to keep the tables simple, statistical tables are generally only horizontal lines and try to avoid using other lines.

The Arabic numbers should be shown on the table, and the number of decimal points retained by the same row or column should be consistent and should be

Table 3.1 The treatment distribution of study

Treatment	Frequency	Percent (%)
Folic acid	66	42.6
Folic acid + iron	42	27.1
Multiple micronutrient	47	30.3
Total	155	100.0

Table 3.2 The treatment distribution of study in two counties

| Treatment | County A | | County B | |
	Frequency	Percent (%)	Frequency	Percent (%)
Folic acid	28	47	38	40
Folic acid + iron	16	27	26	27
Multiple micronutrient	16	27	31	33
Total	60	100	95	100

aligned right. With any missing values labeled ".", usually, "0" indicates a value of zero, and "-" implies no value in that specific cell of the table. There should be no empty cells in the table. Sometimes, the total values are displayed for easy checking or analyzing of the data in the table.

Footnotes should explain all nonstandard abbreviations and other explanations necessary for each table.

3.4   Making Tables Using SPSS

In this chapter, we use a part of data of Study of Impact of Micronutrient Supplementation During Pregnancy on Birthweight as example to show how to make the statistical tables and graphs. There are seven variables of mothers on this dataset such as ID, Treatment (1 = Folic acid, 2 = Folic acid + iron, 3 = Multiple micronutrient), County (1 = County A, 2 = County B), Education (1 = Below and Primary School, 2 = Middle School, 3 = High School and above), Anemia(1 = Yes, 2 = No), Height (cm), and Weight (kg).

Steps of making Table 3.1 using SPSS are as follows:

1. Open the dataset of study.
2. Open the dialog of Frequency shown as Fig. 3.1.
3. Put the variable "treatment" into the right box, and form the table.
4. Obtain the table in the output window of SPSS.

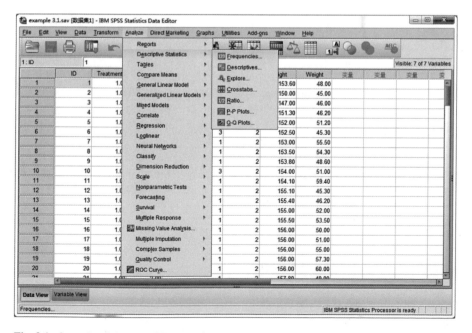

Fig. 3.1 Open the dialogues of Frequencies

5. Copy the table in output, paste to Word, and modify the table to regular statistical table shown as Table 3.1.

Steps of making Table 3.2 using SPSS are as follows:

1. Open the dataset of Study shown.
2. Open the dialog of Crosstabs shown.
3. Put the variable "treatment" into the row box and "County" into the column box from the table.
4. Press the Cell, and select the column in the Percentage box.
5. Obtain the table in the output window of SPSS.
6. Double-click on the table, and change the statistics from row to column.
7. Copy the table in output, paste to Word, and modify the table to regular statistical table shown as Table 3.2.

3.5 Basic Rules and Demands for Graphs

Statistical graphs are also important statistical descriptive methods and can be used to compare and analyze data. Graphs visualize the data as a geometric chart and express the quantitative relationship between the observations or variables by using different notations—the location of a dot, the elevation of a line, the length of a bar, or the size of an area.

An appropriate chart should be chosen to depict the information according to the characteristic of data or the purpose of analyses.

Title: The title should briefly describe the content of the table, which includes the time and place of the observations, and always label a serial number that is located at the top of the table.

Subheadings: The horizontal subheading explains the subject, which is located below the abscissa axis; the vertical subheading shows the predicate, which is located at the left of vertical axis. Abscissas and ordinates should be clearly marked with appropriate units, with the scale labeled from left to right, bottom to top, and small to big. The ratio of the length to the width should be 7:5.

Legends: Different colors or lines can be used to distinguish different data, and they should be labeled by legend. Legends display the main contents of a graph and are located blank of the chart or graph. They should be brief and concise.

3.6 Types of Common Charts

There are many ways to present data in plots, graphs, or charts. Here, we list the ten most common types of charts for categorical and continuous data, as well as their applications.

3.6.1   Bar Chart

A bar chart contains rectangular bars. The bar lengths are proportional to the values that they represent. They can be plotted either vertically or horizontally, although a vertical bar chart is more common. In a vertical bar chart, the group variable is plotted on the *x*-axis, and the frequency variable is plotted on the *y*-axis. The bars should be of equal width and should be separated from one another so as not to imply continuity. The width of the spaces between the bars should be equal to or are half width of a rectangular bar. Furthermore, the spaces should also be equal in width to each other. As usual, the values that are compared would be arranged by numerical order or another natural order for an easy and clear comparison. Bar charts include a simple bar chart, a double bar chart, a stacked bar chart, and a percentage bar chart. Bar charts are used to display a frequency distribution for nominal and ordinal data. The following illustrates how to construct bars using SPSS.

3.6.1.1   A Simple Bar Chart

A simple bar chart was created to display the education distribution of the mothers of the study shown in Fig. 3.2.

Steps of making the simple bar chart using SPSS:

1. Open the dataset of Study.
2. Open the dialog of Bar shown as Fig. 3.3.
3. Select the "Simple" in main dialog of Bar charts.

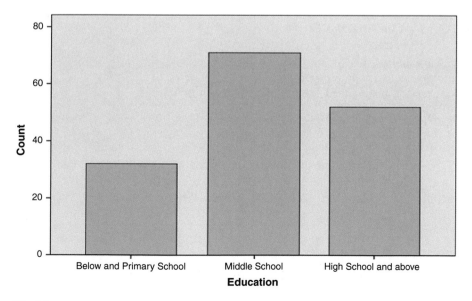

Fig. 3.2 10 Mothers' education distribution

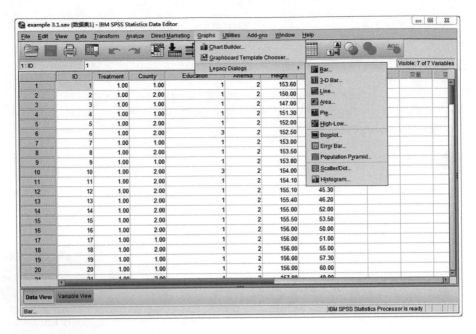

Fig. 3.3 Open the dialog of Bar

4. Select the "education" into Categorical Axis box in the dialog of Define Simple Bar.
5. Obtain the Bar chart in the output window of SPSS.

3.6.1.2 Clustered Bar Chart

A clustered bar chart was constructed to display the education distribution of the mothers in two counties shown in Fig. 3.4.

Steps of making the Clustered Bar Chart using SPSS:

1. Open the dataset of Study.
2. Open the dialog of Bar shown as Fig. 3.3.
3. Select the "Clustered" in main dialog of Bar Charts.
4. Select the "Education" into Categorical Axis box and "Anemia" into "Define Clusters by:" box in the dialog of Define Clustered Bar.
5. Obtain the Simple Bar Chart in the output window of SPSS.

3.6.1.3 Stacked Bar Chart

The relationship between the Education and the County can also be displayed in a Stacked Bar Chart using SPSS shown in Fig. 3.5.

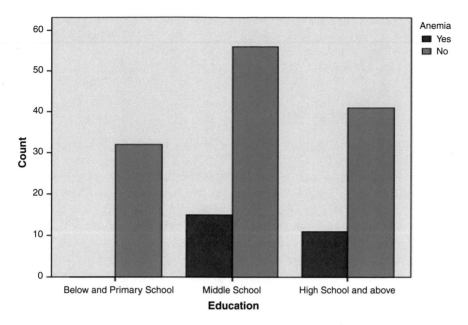

Fig. 3.4 The education distribution of the mothers in two counties

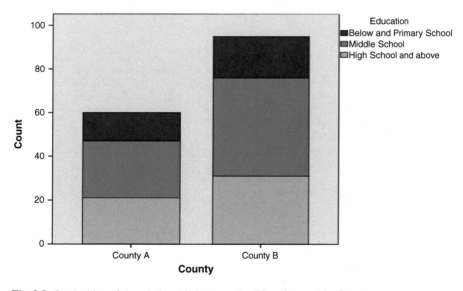

Fig. 3.5 Stacked bar of the relationship between the Education and the County

Steps of making the Stacked Bar Chart using SPSS:

1. Open the dataset of Study.
2. Open the dialog of Bar shown as Fig. 3.3.

3. Select the "Stacked" in main dialog of Bar Charts.
4. Select the "Education" into Categorical Axis box and "County" into "Define Clusters by:" box in the dialog of Define Clustered Bar.
5. Obtain the Simple Bar Chart in the output window of SPSS.

3.6.1.4   Percentage Bar Chart

A percentage bar chart can be used to represent the percentiles of categorical data. It can be made for the above examples from SPSS, if "% of cases" is chosen in bars present of charts dialog box. In such a way, the values in each category of "clustered" or "stacked" variable that you put in the box of "Define Clusters by" or "Define Stacks by" in charts dialog box are summed up to 100%. If a percent bar chart with 100% by each category of "category" variable in the above example, it cannot be generated directly using SPSS; a count stacked bar chart must be edited to create this percentage bar chart. For example, the relationship between the Education and County can also be plotted in a percentage bar chart. First, put the stacked bar chart in the "output" window, choose the stacked bar chart, and double-click the left mouse button to get the Chart Editor.

In Chart Editor window, select "Scale to 100%" on the bottom of Option in Fig. 3.6, and then change the y-axis to percentile on the Chart Editor. Click the "Percent" site, then add "(%)," and change "Percent" into "Percent (%)."

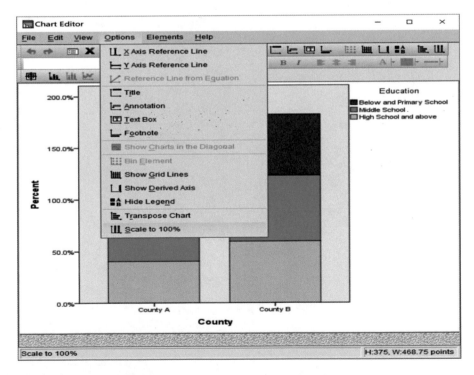

Fig. 3.6 Properties dialog box

3.6.2   Histograms

A histogram is a graph that displays the frequency distribution of a variable for continuous or discrete data. The horizontal axis displays the true limits of the various intervals. The true limits of an interval are the points that separate it from the intervals on either side. The vertical axis of a histogram depicts either the frequency or the relative frequency of observations within each interval. The vertical scale should begin at zero; if it does not, visual comparisons among the intervals may be distorted (Fig. 3.7).

Steps of making the histogram using SPSS:

1. Open the dataset of Study.
2. Open the dialog of Histogram.
3. Move the "Height" into Variable box, and select "display the normal curve."
4. Obtain the histogram in the output window of SPSS.

3.6.3   Stem-and-Leaf Plot

A stem-and-leaf plot is a useful tool in exploratory quantitative data, similar to a histogram. A stem-and-leaf plot shows the spread and distribution of variable's values. Figure 3.8 shows the stem-and-leaf plot of height of study; the left column of dots contains the stems; and the right column of dots contains the leaves. Stems

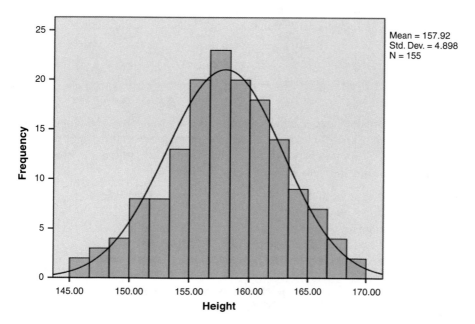

Fig. 3.7 Histogram of height of mother in the study

Fig. 3.8 The stem-and-leaf plot in the output window of SPSS

Height(cm)

Height(cm) Stem-and-Leaf Plot

```
Frequency     Stem &  Leaf

     1.00 Extremes      (=<145)
      .00         14 .
     3.00         14 .  677
     5.00         14 .  88999
     8.00         15 .  00001111
    15.00         15 .  222223333333333
    15.00         15 .  444444555555555
    23.00         15 .  66666666666677777777777
    31.00         15 .  8888888888888888888899999999999
    18.00         16 .  000000000000011111
    15.00         16 .  222222222333333
    14.00         16 .  44444444555555
     4.00         16 .  6777
     3.00         16 .  889

Stem width:      10.00
Each leaf:        1 case(s)
```

represent the first two digits of the value; Frequency represents the number of values with that first two digits. Leaves represent the third digit in the values (numbers 0–9).

Steps of making the stem-and-leaf plot using SPSS:

1. Open the dataset of Study.
2. Open the dialog of Explore.
3. Move the "Height" into Dependent List box.
4. Obtain the Stem-and-Leaf Plot in the output window of SPSS shown as Fig. 3.8.

3.6.4   Pie Chart

A pie chart is mainly used to show the proportion of each slice. The total area of a circular chart is 100%; the area of each slice is proportional to the quantity it represents. Figure 3.9 is a pie chart showing the education's proportion of mothers.

Steps of making the stem-and-leaf plot using SPSS:

1. Open the dataset of Study.
2. Open the dialog of Pie.
3. Select "Summaries for groups of cases" in Pie Charts dialog.
4. Move the "Education" into "Define Slices by:" box.
5. Choose the pie chart, and double-click the left mouse button in the Chart Editor Window.
6. Click the right mouse button, choose "Show Data Labels," and obtain the Pie Chart in the output window of SPSS shown as Fig. 3.9.

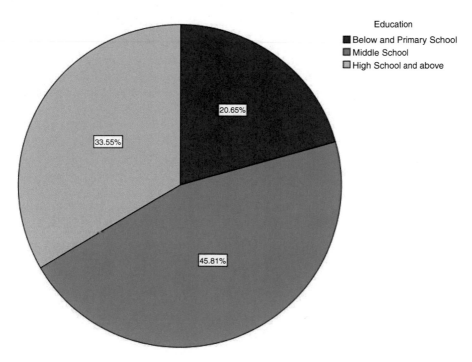

Fig. 3.9 Pie chart of mothers' educational proportion

3.6.5 *Line Chart*

A line chart or line graph displays information as a series of data points connected by straight line segments. It can be used to illustrate the relationship between continuous quantities. The variable of time or concentration is usually labeled on the *x*-axis, while count or rate is on the *y*-axis. Each value on the *x*-axis has a single corresponding measurement on the *y*-axis. Adjacent points are connected by a straight line.

Line charts can be divided into two types—common line charts and semilogarithmic line charts. When composing a common line graph, the scale must be an arithmetic scale on both the *x*- and *y*-axes. A series of points that represent individual measurements must be connected by line segments. A common line chart is often used to visualize the magnitude of changes in data over intervals of time or concentration.

When drawing a semilogarithmic line chart, the *y*-axis scale is logarithmic, while the *x*-axis scale remains arithmetic. The series of points should still be connected by line segments. Semilogarithmic line charts are suitable for visualizing the count or rate of change in a variable over time or concentration.

A line chart is an extension of a scatter plot. For example, Table 3.3 displays the mortality of diarrhea and pertussis in a certain place between 1975 and 2000. A common line chart is used to describe trends in mortality of diarrhea and pertussis over time shown in Fig. 3.10; a semilogarithmic line chart is suitable for showing the rate of mortality of diarrhea and pertussis over time shown in Fig. 3.11.

To construct a common line chart using data in Table 3.3, the SPSS steps are as follows:

1. Open the dataset of Table 3.3, and then open the dialog of Line.
2. Select "Multiple" and "Summaries of separate variables" in the Line Charts.
3. Move "mortality of diarrhea" and "mortality of pertussis" into "Lines Represent:" box, and "Year" into "Category Axis."
4. Double-click on the Line Charts; open a Chart Editor; click the Add Markers; add the markers of two lines; and change the "Mean" into "Mortality (1/10000000)" shown as Fig. 3.10.

Table 3.3 The mortality of diarrhea and pertussis in a certain place between 1975 and 2000

Year	Mortality of diarrhea (1/10,000,000)	Mortality of pertussis (1/10,000,000)
1975	14.5	2.8
1980	9.5	1.6
1985	3.7	0.9
1990	1.6	0.4
1995	0.7	0.2
2000	0.4	0.1

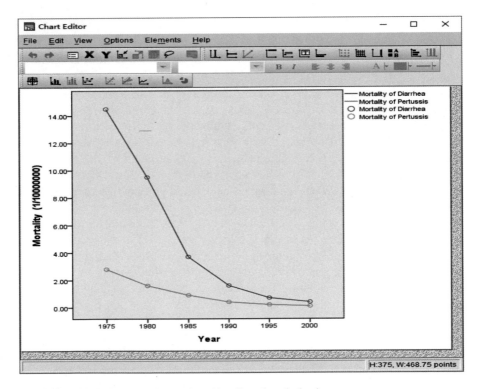

Fig. 3.10 Add markers and change the subheading of vertical axis

5. Close the window.
6. Obtain the Line Chart in the output window of SPSS.

Steps for a semilogarithmic line chart:

1. Open the dataset of Table 3.3, and then open the dialog of Compute Variable as Fig. 3.11.
2. Select "Arithmetic" in the "Function group" box, and move "Lg10" from the "Functions and Special Variables:" box into "Numeric Expression" box, and then put "Diarrhea" into parentheses replace the "?".
3. Name the variable in "Target Variable:" box, then click "Type & Label," and define the Label of Target Variable.
4. Compute the Lg10 of "Pertussis" as the same way as "Diarrhea."
5. Obtain the semilogarithmic line chart in the output window of SPSS in the same way.

3.6.6 Scatter Plot

Scatter plots are often useful graphs for understanding the relationship between two or more different continuous measurements that are measured in a group. They are very important tools in correlation and regression analysis in statistics.

There are four scatter plots in SPSS: The one-way scatter plot uses a single horizontal axis to display the relative position of each data point; the matrix scatter plot

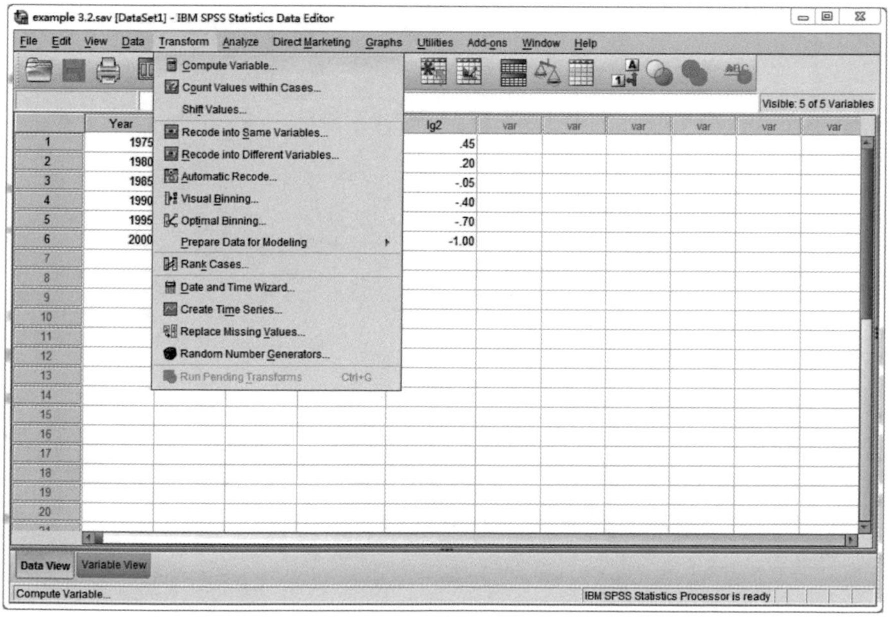

Fig. 3.11 Open the dataset and the dialog of Compute Variable

is used to depict the relationship between multiple variables; an overlay scatter is suitable for showing the relationship among multiple independent variables and one dependent variable, or multiple dependent variables and one independent variable; a 3-D scatter is used to express the integral relationship among three variables.

Figure 3.12 shows the simple scatter plot of the height (cm) and weight (kg) of mothers in the study. Each circle on this graph shows the height and weight of a study subject.

Steps of making the simple scatter plot using SPSS:

1. Open the dataset of Study and the dialog of Scatter/Dot.
2. Select "Simple Scatter" in the dialog of Scatter/Dot.
3. Move the "Height" as variable X into "X Axis" box and the "Weight" as variable Y into "Y Axis" box.
4. Obtain the Simple Scatter Chart in the output window of SPSS shown as Fig. 3.11.

3.6.7 Box Plot

A box plot (also called a box-and-whiskers plot) is a way of summarizing data using five statistics—minimum, first quartile (Q1, known as the 25th percentile), median (second quartile (Q2), the 50th percentile), third quartile (Q3, 75th percentile), and

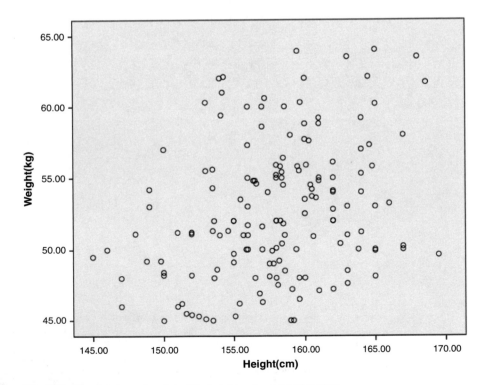

Fig. 3.12 The simple scatter plot of the height and weight of mothers

maximum—to give a basic representation of the structure of data. Box plots can also roughly show the dispersion of the data distribution (especially useful for comparing several samples) and whether the data are symmetrical.

Figure 3.12 shows such plots for the height of mothers in two counties. In each plot, the thick black line in the middle of the box marks the median; the sides of the box mark the 25th and 75th percentiles, which are also called the first and third quartiles. The width of the box is known as the interquartile range (IQR). The middle 50% of the observations lie within this range. The whiskers extend on either side of the box. The horizontal bars at the end of each whisker mark the most extreme observations that are not more than 1.5 times the IQR from their adjacent quartiles. Any values beyond these bars are plotted separately as a dot plot; these values are called outliers (extreme values). The observations that are more than 1.5 times the IQR are called mild outliers, labeled as "●"; the observations that are more than 3 times the IQR are called extreme outliers, labeled as "*". The outliers merit special consideration, because they may have undue influence on some of the analyses.

As one of many statistical tools, the box plot has unique features. Other than identifying outliers straightforwardly, it can also determine the skew and tail weight of data. Datasets in which the observations are more stretched out on one side of the median than the other are called skewed. They are skewed to the right, if values above the median are more dispersed than are values below; they are skewed to the left when the converse is true. Box plots are particularly valuable when a comparison of the distributions of a variable in different groups is desired.

Steps of making the Box plot using SPSS:

1. Open the dataset of Study and the dialog of Box plot.
2. Select "Simple" in the dialog of Box plot.
3. Move the "Height" into "Variables" box and the "County" into "Category Axis" box.
4. Obtain the Simple Scatter Chart in the output window of SPSS shown as Fig. 3.13.

3.6.8 Mean and Standard Error Chart

The mean and standard error chart is sometimes also referred to as an error bar. A box plot is used to show the distribution of the data, while an error bar displays the population that the data come from and estimates the dispersion of the data. Like box plot, error bars also show the observation summary or single variable summary using three statistics of confidence interval, standard deviation, and standard error. Figure 3.14 shows the 95% confidence intervals of height of mothers based on treatment in an error bar. It gives a general idea of how accurate a measurement is, or conversely, how far from the reported value the true (error free) value might be.

Steps of making the mean and standard error chart using SPSS:

1. Open the dataset of Study and the dialog of Error Bar 1.
2. Select "Simple" in the dialog of Error Bar 1.

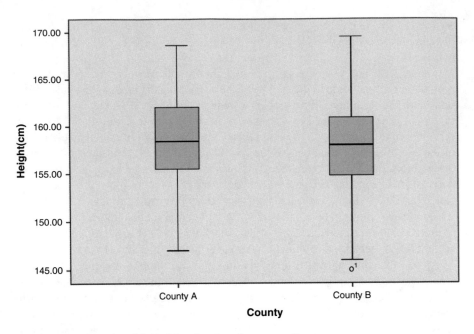

Fig. 3.13 The box plot of the height of mothers in two counties

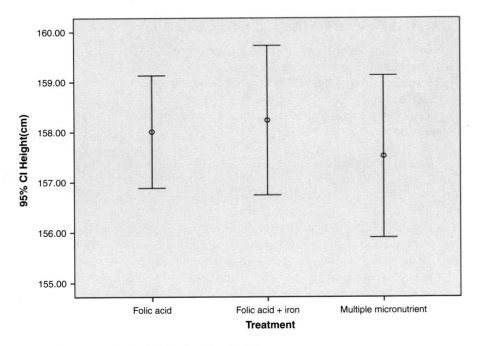

Fig. 3.14 The error bar for height of mothers in different treatments

3. Move the "Height" into "Variables" box and the "Treatment" into "Category Axis" box 1.
4. Obtain the Simple Scatter Chart in the output window of SPSS.

Chapter Summary

1. The statistical results presented in a table include title, row and column headings, straight lines, numbers, and, if necessary, notes; A table is usually recommended for three horizontal lines: cap line, line between, and bottom line.
2. The common graphs include bar charts, histograms, stem-and-leaf plot, pie charts, line graphs, scatter plots, box plots, and mean and standard error chart. Table 3.4 summarizes purposes and illustrations of graphs (Table 3.4).

Table 3.4 Purposes and illustrations of graphs

Types	Applications	Purposes	Illustrations
Bar chart	Continuous or discrete data	To compare the indicators of independent groups	One axis shows group names; the other one shows the value of indicator. A legend is necessary when there are two or more indicators in one chart
Percentage bar chart	Discrete data	To compare the proportions of two group	One axis shows variable names; the scale of the other one is 0% to 100%. The legend must be added to distinguish all elements
Histogram	Continuous data	To describe the frequency distribution	The horizontal axis displays the true limits of the intervals into which the observations fall; the vertical axis depicts the frequency or relative frequency of observations within each interval
Stem-and-leaf plot	Continuous data	Show the spread and distribution of variable's values	A stem-and-leaf plot is a useful tool. Stems represent the first two digits of the value; leaves represent the third digit in the values
Pie chart	Discrete data	To describe the proportion	No axes. A legend must be added to distinguish all elements
Line chart	Continuous data	To illustrate the relationship between two continuous measurements	There is a one-to-one relationship between two variables, with the horizontal axis for the independent variable and the vertical axis for the dependent variable
Semilogarithmic line chart	Continuous data	Same as line chart	It is drawn when the dependent variable has great variability
Box plot	Continuous or discrete data	To display a summary of the observations	It uses a single vertical or horizontal axis
Scatter plot	Continuous data	To describe the relationship between two variables	There may not be a one-to-one relationship between two variables; the horizontal axis shows the independent variable, and the vertical axis shows the dependent variable
Mean and standard error chart	Continuous or discrete data	To show the observation summary or single variable summary	Using three statistics of confidence interval, standard deviation, and standard error

Chapter 4
Descriptive Statistics of Continuous Variables

Lijuan Wu and Chanjuan Zhao

Objectives

Two main components of classical statistical methods are descriptive statistics and inferential statistics. Descriptive statistics describe the main features of a collection of data quantitatively. Their purpose is to describe a distribution of a property, the measure of central tendency, and the dispersion of a very large or infinite population. The normal distribution in particular is discussed in this chapter.

Key Concepts

Descriptive statistics; Continuous variable; Distribution; Normal distribution

4.1 Introduction

Descriptive statistics describe the main features of a collection of data quantitatively. They provide simple summaries about the sample. If the height of students in a course is measured, the height varies continuously. An attempt to capture the full meaning of "student height" in a few numbers is bound to fail—nature is much more complex than a statistical description of it. Researchers need to get the height

L. Wu (✉)
School of Public Health, Capital Medical University, Beijing, China

C. Zhao
School of Public Health, Hainan Medical University, Haikou, China

© Zhengzhou University Press 2024
X. Guo, F. Xue (eds.), *Textbook of Medical Statistics*,
https://doi.org/10.1007/978-981-99-7390-3_4

of every student in the course or the height in a representative sample. They therefore need to describe the central tendency and variation of measurements of the
height. This chapter introduces several statistics which are commonly used to
describe the distribution of data.

4.2 Distribution

4.2.1 Frequency Table

A distribution is a summary of the frequency of a range of values for a variable. The
simplest distribution is a frequency distribution, which lists the frequency of every
value of a variable.

A frequency distribution shows the number of observations falling into each of
several ranges of values and is portrayed as frequency tables and histograms.

A frequency table is one type of table that lists the frequencies of various intervals of values. A frequency table displays data in a clear and easy way to understand.

Example 4.1 The body mass index (BMI) of 100 students aged 6 to 17 years were
recorded to the nearest kilogram per meter^2.

15.7	**21.0**	15.6	14.1	15.4	13.7	15.6	17.4	19.0	16.1
17.6	17.0	16.4	17.3	17.3	17.6	14.6	14.3	17.4	16.0
15.0	18.1	18.1	19.6	20.1	19.0	15.1	19.0	19.8	16.8
15.6	19.2	14.4	16.9	17.8	15.2	16.0	19.4	14.7	18.2
18.0	16.6	18.3	18.6	16.6	17.1	15.7	17.9	16.0	16.0
17.3	18.1	17.6	14.0	16.3	18.9	**13.6**	20.9	16.8	14.3
17.8	18.7	14.8	17.9	17.8	17.6	18.7	15.2	19.0	16.0
14.4	17.1	17.1	16.4	17.0	15.1	17.4	16.7	17.1	16.7
16.6	16.1	17.6	19.2	15.7	15.6	14.5	16.3	18.9	14.9
17.6	19.7	16.3	15.4	16.0	18.1	17.4	15.6	14.3	19.1

The observations were then subdivided into intervals of equal width, and the
frequencies corresponding to each interval are presented in Table 4.1.

Table 4.1 provides an overall picture of what the data look like; it shows how the
values of BMI are distributed across the intervals. Note that the observations range
from 13.6 to 21.0 kg/m^2, with relatively few measurements in the first or last few
intervals and a large proportion of values falling into intervals between 15.4 and
18.6 kg/m^2. The interval of 17.0 to <17.8 kg/m^2 contains the largest number of
observations.

The following steps describe how to construct a frequency table. First, scan the
raw data to determine the range of values, which extends from 13.6 to 21.0 kg/m^2.
The range is 21.0–13.6 = 7.4 kg/m^2.

Table 4.1 Absolute frequencies of BMI in 100 students aged 6 to 17 years

BMI (kg/m^2)	Number of subjects
13.0~	2
13.8~	8
14.6~	9
15.4~	18
16.2~	13
17.0~	19
17.8~	12
18.6~	12
19.4~	5
20.2 ~ 21.0	2

Second, choose the appropriate intervals for a tally. If there are too many intervals, the summary is not much of an improvement over the raw data; too few intervals, a great deal of information is lost; 8 to 15 intervals are appropriate with 100 observations.

The width of each interval is computed by dividing the number of intervals by the range of values. In Table 4.1, the interval width is $(21.0–13.6)/10 = 0.74$ (kg/m^2). Using interval widths that are both easy to plot and easy to interpret is logical, such as a width of 0.8 (kg/m^2).

In the example above, the first interval between 13.0 and <13.8 indicates that the values go from the value of 13.0 up to but do not include 13.8 kg/m^2 to avoid a possible overlap.

Third, construct a table that consists of the interval of BMI levels, go through the list of BMI values, and count the number for each interval.

The relative frequency for an interval is the proportion of the total number of observations that fall in that interval. It is computed by dividing the number of values within an interval by the total number of values in the table. The proportion can be multiplied by 100% to obtain the percentage of values within the interval. In Table 4.2, the relative frequency in the first interval is $(2/100) \times 100\% = 2\%$; similarly, the relative frequency in the 13.0 to <13.8 kg/m^2 class is $(2/100) \times 100\% = 2\%$.

The cumulative relative frequency for an interval is the percentage of the total number of observations that have a value less than or equal to the upper limit of that interval. The cumulative relative frequency is calculated by adding up the relative frequency for the specified interval and all previous intervals.

4.2.2 Characteristics of Distribution

For continuous data, the characteristics of distribution displayed by frequency table or graphs could be summarized in four aspects:

Table 4.2 Relative and cumulative relative frequencies of BMI levels for 100 students aged 6 to 17 years

BMI (kg/m²)	Number of subjects	Relative frequency (%)	Cumulative relative frequency (%)
13.0~	2	2	2
13.8~	8	8	10
14.6~	9	9	19
15.4~	18	18	37
16.2~	13	13	50
17.0~	19	19	69
17.8~	12	12	81
18.6~	12	12	93
19.4~	5	5	98
20.2 ~ 21.0	2	2	100

1. Shape: Why do we care about the shape? That is because many statistical methods assume the shape is symmetric and bell shaped (Normal distribution), and these methods are not appropriate if the distribution is skewed.
2. Location: Another expression of central tendency or center, which could be measured by mean, median, mode.
3. Spread: Also known as spread or variability, which could be measured by range, interquartile range (IQR), standard deviation, and variance.
4. Unusual data value: The outlier, showing an extreme deviation from the center, and sometimes with valuable information in medical practice.

4.2.3   Types of Distribution

Every textbook of statistics provides a listing of statistical distributions, with their properties, but browsing through these choices can be frustrating to anyone without a statistical background. When analyzing continuous data and trying to fit the right distribution to that data, we need to look at:

1. Symmetry: There are some data sets that exhibit symmetry, i.e., the upside is mirrored by the downside, or the left side is mirrored by the right side. The symmetric distribution that most practitioners have familiarity with is the normal distribution; see Fig. 4.1a–c.
2. Skews: Most data does not exhibit symmetry and instead skews toward either very large positive or very large negative values. If the data is positively skewed, the distribution lies in the right direction; see Fig. 4.2a. If the data is negatively skewed, the distribution lies in the left direction; see Fig. 4.2b.

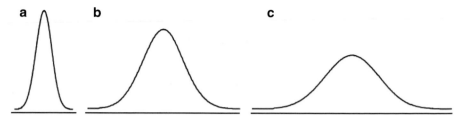

Fig. 4.1 (a–c) Symmetric distribution

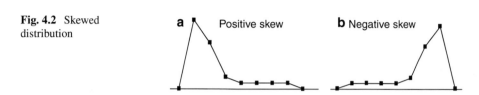

Fig. 4.2 Skewed distribution

4.3 Measures of Location

The most commonly investigated characteristic of a set of data is the center, the point around which the observations tend to cluster.

4.3.1 Arithmetic Mean

The arithmetic mean is simply called the "mean" that is calculated by adding all the observations in a set of data and then dividing the sum by the total number of measures. The average of all of the values in a population is defined as the population mean, denoted by the Greek letter μ. In statistics, μ is usually unavailable, so information about the population mean μ is gathered from sample mean $\bar{X}$. Many normal distributions are best described by their mean.

The sample mean $\bar{X}$ of observations $X_1, X_2\ldots, X_n$ is defined as:

$$\bar{X} = \frac{X_1 + X_2 +, \ldots, X_n}{n} = \frac{\sum_{i=1}^{n} x_i}{n} \tag{4.1}$$

Example 4.2 If the values of creatinine clearances for the $n = 5$ male transplant patients are as follow: 38, 66, 74, 99, and 80, then

$$\bar{X} = \frac{38 + 66 + 74 + 99 + 80}{5} = 71.4.$$

For the grouped data,

$$\bar{X} = \frac{\sum f_i X_i}{\sum f_i} = \frac{\sum f_i X_i}{n} \tag{4.2}$$

where f_i refers to the frequencies corresponding to each interval and X_i refers to the mid-value of the class.

4.3.2 Geometric Mean

The geometric mean indicates the central tendency or typical value of a set of numbers which are multiplied, with the nth root of the resulting product taken.

$$G = \sqrt[n]{X_1 X_2 \ldots X_n} = \log^{-1}\left(\frac{\sum_{i=1}^{n} \log X_i}{n}\right) \tag{4.3}$$

The latter expression states that the log of the geometric mean is the arithmetic mean of the logs of the numbers. The geometric mean only applies to positive numbers. It is also often used for a set of numbers whose values are meant to be multiplied together or are exponential in nature, such as data on human population growth or interest rates of a financial investment.

Example 4.3 Find the geometric mean of the values 10, 100, 1000, 10,000, 100,000.

lgG = (lg10 + lg100 + lg1000 + lg10000 + lg100000)/5 = (1 + 2 + 3 + 4 + 5)/5 = 3.

$G = 10^3 = 1000$.

If there are a series of n positive values with repeated values, such as $X_1, X_2, \ldots, X_k$ repeated $f_1, f_2, \ldots, f_k$ times, respectively, then the geometric mean becomes:

$$G = \log^{-1}\left(\frac{\sum f_i \log X_i}{\sum f_i}\right) \tag{4.4}$$

4.3.3 Median

The *median* of a finite list of numbers can be found by arranging all the observations from the lowest value to the highest value and choosing the middle value.

If n is odd, M is equal to the $\left(\dfrac{n+1}{2}\right)^{th}$ ordered value.

If n is even, M is equal to the average of $\left(\dfrac{n}{2}\right)^{th}$ and $\left(\dfrac{n}{2}+1\right)^{th}$ ordered value.

Example 4.4 A rank ordering of a group of observations ($n = 23$) from lowest to highest would produce the following:

$$1,2,2,3,3,3,4,4,4,5,5,\underline{5},5,5,5,6,6,6,6,7,7,7,8,8.$$

In this case, 5 (the 12th ordered value) is the median, which is the value that falls in the exact center of the distribution. If one more observation (20) is added, then the median (represented by an underlined area) is located between the two center values (12 data points are above and 12 data points are below this center):

$$1,2,2,3,3,3,4,4,4,5,5,5,\_5,5,6,6,6,6,7,7,7,8,8,20.$$

The calculation of the median would be:

$$(5+5)/2 = 5.$$

The calculation of the median of grouped data is based on the following formula:

$$M = L_M + \frac{i}{f_M}\left(n \times 50\% - \Sigma\, fL\right) \tag{4.5}$$

L_M = the lower limit of the class containing the median. n = the total number of frequencies.

f_M = the frequency of the median class

ΣfL = the cumulative number of frequencies in the classes preceding the class containing the median

i = the width of the class containing the median.

Example 4.5 In Table 4.2, the median contained in the fifth class (16.2~) is given by:

$$M = L_M + \frac{i}{f_M}\left(n \times 50\% - \Sigma\, fL\right) = 16.2 + \frac{0.8}{13}\left(100 \times 50\% - 37\right) = 17.0$$

If data is normally distributed, or the sample is assumed to be drawn from a normally distributed population, the mean is the best measure of central tendency. The median is the preferred measure of central tendency in skewed distributions where there are a few extreme values (either small or large).

4.4 Measures of Variation

The mean and median describe the central tendency of the observations; they do not tell the whole story of a data set. In medical practice, individuals vary physiologically, biochemically, and in response to disease or treatments. Variations occur both within subjects and between subjects. Some of the variation can be explained by known causes, such as age, gender, etc., but there are also unknown causes of variation. Thus, another characteristic of a data set is its variation due to the spread of the observations.

4.4.1 Range

The range is defined as the difference between the highest and the lowest values of the data. It considers only the extreme values of a data set instead of the majority of the observations. Although it is useful, it is too crude for a measure of variability. For instance, we would describe the "spread" of these numbers: 18, 19, 20, 21, and 22 as range = 22–18 = 4.

4.4.2 Interquartile Range

In statistics, a **percentile** (or centile) is the value of a variable below which a certain percentage of observations fall. For example, the 15th percentile is the value (or score) below which 15% of the observations may be found.

The 25th percentile is also known as the first quartile (Q_1), the 50th percentile as the median or the second quartile (Q_2), and the 75th percentile as the third quartile (Q_3).

Therefore, the interquartile range is calculated by subtracting the 25th percentile from the 75th percentile of the data. Consequently, it encompasses the middle 50% of the observations.

Interquartile range is robust to extreme values; therefore, it is commonly used in describing the variation of distribution free data.

4.4.3   Variance and Standard Deviation

The variance quantifies the amount of variability, or spread, around the mean of the measurements. The average distance of the individual observations from the sample mean can be calculated:

$$\Sigma\left(X_i - \bar{X}\right).$$

However, it can be shown mathematically that $\Sigma\left(X_i - \bar{X}\right)$ is always equal to zero. To solve this problem, a more widely used procedure is to square the deviations.

$$SS = \Sigma\left(X_i - \bar{X}\right)^2 \tag{4.6}$$

More explicitly, the variance is calculated by subtracting the mean of a set of values from each of the observations, squaring these deviations, adding them up, and then dividing the resulting number by 1 less than the number of observations in the data set. The variance is represented by S^2.

$$S^2 = \frac{\sum\limits_{i=1}^{n}\left(X_i - \bar{X}\right)^2}{n-1} \tag{4.7}$$

Example 4.6 If a sample of observations [1, 5, 7, 8, 79] with sample mean as 20, the variance is

$$
\begin{aligned}
S^2 &= \frac{(1-20)^2 + (5-20)^2 + (7-20)^2 + (8-20)^2 + (79-20)^2}{5-1}\\[2mm]
&= \frac{(-19)^2 + (-15)^2 + (-13)^2 + (-12)^2 + (59)^2}{5-1}\\[2mm]
&= \frac{361 + 225 + 169 + 144 + 3481}{4} = \frac{4380}{4} = 1095
\end{aligned}
$$

The standard deviation of a set of data is the positive square root of the variance. Thus, for the five measurements above, the standard deviation is equal to:

$$S = \sqrt{S^2} = \sqrt{1095} = 33.09.$$

Variance is not as easily interpreted, because it is measured in square units instead of the original units of measurement; thus in practice, the standard deviation is used more frequently. Both of variance and standard deviation measure the "average" distance of data points from the mean using all the data values, especially appropriate for normal distributed data.

4.4.4   Coefficient of Variation

The coefficient of variation, a measurement of relative variability, relates the standard deviation of a set of values to its mean—it is the ratio of S to $\bar{X}$ multiplied by 100%. The coefficient of variation is a dimensionless number because of sharing the same measurement unit of the standard deviation and mean. The coefficient of variation can be used to compare the variability among two or more sets of data representing different quantities and different units of measurement.

$$CV = \frac{S}{\bar{X}} \times 100\% \tag{4.8}$$

A data set of [100, 100, 100] has constant values. Its standard deviation is 0, and average is 100, giving the coefficient of variation as 0/100 = 0.

A data set of [90, 100,110] has more variability. Its standard deviation is 10, and its average is 100, giving the coefficient of variation as 10/100 = 0.1.

4.5   Normal Distribution

The most common continuous distribution is the normal distribution, also known as the Gaussian distribution or the bell-shaped curve. It is often used as an initial approximation to describe real-valued random variables that tend to cluster around a single mean value. Its probability density is given by the equation:

$$f(x) = \frac{1}{\sigma\sqrt{2\pi}} e^{\frac{-(x-\mu)^2}{2\sigma^2}} \tag{4.9}$$

where $-\infty < X < \infty$; the symbol π is a constant of 3.14 (Fig. 4.3).

4.5.1   Characteristics of the Normal Distribution

1. The normal curve is unimodal and symmetric about its mean, μ (mju).
2. The standard deviation, represented by σ (sigma), specifies the amount of dispersion around the mean. Together, the two parameters of μ and σ completely define a normal curve. The notation $N(\mu, \sigma^2)$ means that the data are normally distributed with mean μ and variance σ^2, expressed as $X \sim N(\mu, \sigma^2)$.
3. The total area under the normal curve is equal to 1. The area under the curve between $\mu - 1*SD$ and $\mu + 1*SD$ is 68.27%; the area under the curve between $\mu - 1.96*SD$ and $\mu + 1.96*SD$ is 95%; and the area under the curve between $\mu - 2.58*SD$ and $\mu + 2.58*SD$ is 99% (Fig. 4.4).

Fig. 4.3 The normal curve

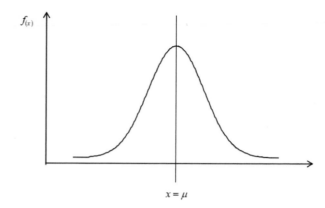

Fig. 4.4 The area under
normal curve

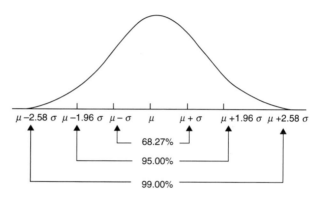

4.5.2 The Standard Normal Distribution

Since a normal distribution could have an infinite number of possible values for its
mean and standard deviation, it is impossible to tabulate the area associated with
each normal curve. Instead, only a single curve is tabulated—the special case for
which $\mu = 0$ and $\sigma = 1$. This curve is referred to as the standard normal distribution.
The standard normal distribution of Z Table in appendix displays the areas in the
upper tail of the standard normal distribution. The integer number and tenths decimal places of Z are listed in the left column of the table, and the hundreds decimal
places are listed across the top row. For a particular value of Z, the entry in the table
specifies the area beneath the curve to the right of z.

   In other words, a problem involving a normally distributed variable X with mean
μ and standard deviation σ is not solved directly. Instead, the problem is converted
into an equivalent problem that deals with a normal variable measured in standardized deviation units, called a standardized normal variable (Z). For instance, if $X \sim N$
$(\mu, \sigma2)$, then

$$Z = \frac{X - \mu}{\sigma} \sim N(0,1) \tag{4.10}$$

Fig. 4.5 The standard
normal curve

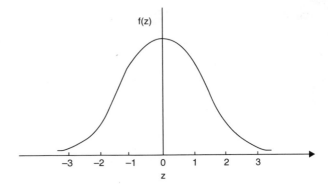

Probabilities could be tabulated for a single distribution and used to address problems using any other normal distribution. We can a.o compare observations from two different normal distributions or distributions with different original units because the units of Z-score are standard deviations (Fig. 4.5).

4.5.3　Application of Normal Distribution

Many naturally occurring random processes tend to have a distribution that is approximately normal. The normal distribution is the most widely used continuous distribution. Thus, because of its omnipresence, the normal distribution is vital to statistical work, most estimation procedures, and hypothesis tests. Another important area of application of the normal distribution is as an approximating distribution to other distributions. Also, the percentiles of a normal distribution are often referred to as statistical inference. The followings are the three of the common and useful applications for the normal distribution.

1. Calculating Probabilities Using the Normal Distribution

    To determine probabilities involving a normal distribution, use the following procedure. A calculating device or a table is needed to obtain an answer.

    (a) Step 1: Formulate question in mathematical terms by putting it into the $P(X < z)$ form.
    (b) Step 2: Standardize any values to a z-score by subtracting the mean and dividing the difference by the standard deviation (i.e., use $Z = (X - \mu)/\sigma$).
    (c) Step 3: Get probability by looking up your z-scores in the z-table, or use a calculating device. The value in the table is $P(Z < z)$, the probability that the random variable, Z, is less than your calculated z-score.
    (d) Step 4: Answer the question. Since the table only gives $P(Z < z)$, you may have some extra work.

    - To find $P(Z > z)$, subtract the table value from 1.
    - To find $P(a < Z < b)$, subtract $P(Z < a)$ from $P(Z < b)$.

Example 4.7 Assume that birth weights for newborns of gestational age between 38 and 42 weeks are normally distributed with a mean of 3400 g and a standard deviation 700 g. What is the probability that a newborn of gestational age between 38 and 42 weeks will have a birth weight between 2500 and 3500 g?

Solution:

$$z_1 = \frac{2500 - 3400}{700} = -1.29 \Rightarrow P(X > 2500) = P(Z > -1.29) = 1 - P(Z < -1.29)$$
$$= 1 - 0.099 = 0.901$$

$$z_2 = \frac{3500 - 3400}{700} = 0.14 \Rightarrow P(X > 3500) = P(Z > 0.14)$$
$$= P(Z < -0.14) = 0.444$$

$$P(2500 < X < 3500) = P(-1.29 < z < 0.14) = P(Z > -1.29) - P(Z > 0.14)$$
$$= 0.901 - 0.444 = 0.457$$

2. Determining the Measurement Values for x

The Z-table can also be used for the reverse process to find a value for x given a probability reverse the process above.

(a) Step 1: Formulate question into $P(X < x)$ form.
(b) Step 2: Rewrite question if necessary using $P(X > x) = 1 - P(X < x)$.
(c) Step 3: Get Z-score from table, computer, or calculator.
(d) Step 4: Determine x by using the Z-score. Remember $x = \mu + Z\sigma$.

Example 4.8 Assume that birth weights for newborns of gestational age between 38 and 42 weeks are normally distributed with a mean of 3400 g and a standard deviation 700 g. Pediatricians define newborns as "large for gestational age," if their weight is above the 90th percentile for their gestational age. Identify the birth weight above which newborns with gestational age between 38 and 42 weeks would be considered "large for gestational age"? ($Z_{0.1} = 1.28$).

Solution: $x = \mu + Z \cdot \sigma = 3400 + 1.28 \cdot 700 = 4296$

3. Establishing Reference Ranges

In clinical practice, some lab tests provide a simple "yes" or "no" answer. For instance, was the test positive for the bacteria that cause strep throat? Many other tests, however, are reported as numbers or values. Laboratory test results reported as numbers are not meaningful by themselves. Their meaning comes from comparison to reference values. Reference values are the values expected for a healthy person. They are sometimes called "normal" values.

We can calculate 95% reference ranges two ways: using percentiles of the observed data or using the normal distribution. If it is reasonable to assume a normal distribution, the second will give more reliable estimates if the sample is small.

Example 4.9 Birth weights again, for instance, assume that birth weights for 30,000 newborns of gestational age between 38 and 42 weeks are normally distributed with a mean of 3400 g and a standard deviation 700 g. Establish the 95% reference range based on this sample.

Either low birth weight or high birth weight babies may be more at risk for certain health problems, so reference ranges should be estimated in two-sided.

Solution 1: Find the 2.5th percentile and 97.5th percentile such that approximately 95% of 30,000 observed values are within the reference range.

Solution 2: Upper limit

$$\bar{X} + 1.96S = 3400 + 1.96^*700 = 4772 \; (\text{gram})$$

Lower limit

$$\bar{X} - 1.96S = 3400 - 1.96^*700 = 2028 \; (\text{gram})$$

4. Identifying Outliers

Outliers are values that "lie outside" the other values, having the biggest effect on the mean in a data set, and not so much on the median or mode. So if mean is going to be used to summarize the data set central tendency, outliers should be identified and be carefully checked first. Empirically, any value outside of three standard deviations from mean value would be identified as an outlier.

Example 4.10 Assume that birth weights for newborns of gestational age between 38 and 42 weeks are normally distributed with a mean of 3400 g and a standard deviation 700 g. Any newborn of gestational age between 38 and 42 weeks has a birth weight either lower than 3400–3*700 = 1300 (g) or higher than 3400 + 3*700 = 5500 (g) would be considered as an outlier.

4.6 Application

Example 4.11 The body mass index(BMI) of 100 students aged 6 to 17 years were recorded to the nearest kilogram per meter^2.

15.7	**21.0**	15.6	14.1	15.4	13.7	15.6	17.4	19.0	16.1
17.6	17.0	16.4	17.3	17.3	17.6	14.6	14.3	17.4	16.0
15.0	18.1	18.1	19.6	20.1	19.0	15.1	19.0	19.8	16.8
15.6	19.2	14.4	16.9	17.8	15.2	16.0	19.4	14.7	18.2
18.0	16.6	18.3	18.6	16.6	17.1	15.7	17.9	16.0	16.0
17.3	18.1	17.6	14.0	16.3	18.9	**13.6**	20.9	16.8	14.3
17.8	18.7	14.8	17.9	17.8	17.6	18.7	15.2	19.0	16.0
14.4	17.1	17.1	16.4	17.0	15.1	17.4	16.7	17.1	16.7
16.6	16.1	17.6	19.2	15.7	15.6	14.5	16.3	18.9	14.9
17.6	19.7	16.3	15.4	16.0	18.1	17.4	15.6	14.3	19.1

4.6.1   Opening a SPSS Data File

The data in this example were inputted into SPSS: File → Open → Data → select the data location.

4.6.2   Conducting a Normality Test Using SPSS

The main process for conducting a normality test using SPSS 20.0 is:

Analyze → Non-parametric Test → One-sample KS → enter *BMI* in the test variable list → OK.

Step by step process:

1. Analyze → Nonparametric Test → One-sample KS (as shown in Fig. 4.6).
2. In the One-sample KS dialog box, enter *BMI* in the test variable list → select OK.
3. SPSS Outcome.

Figure 4.7 shows the main outcomes of the normality test: $Z = 0.474$ and $P = 0.978 > 0.05$, so H_0 cannot be rejected and the data follow a normal distribution.

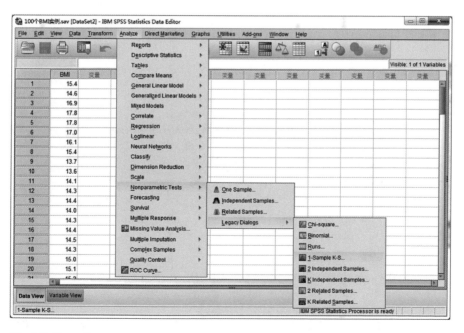

Fig. 4.6 Normality test

Fig. 4.7 Outcome of the normality test

One-Sample Kolmogorov-Smirnov Test

		BMI
N		100
Normal Parameters[a,b]	Mean	16.892
	Std. Deviation	1.6766
Most Extreme Differences	Absolute	.047
	Positive	.047
	Negative	-.045
Kolmogorov-Smirnov Z		.474
Asymp. Sig. (2-tailed)		.978

a. Test distribution is Normal.

b. Calculated from data.

Fig. 4.8 SPSS Outcome

Descriptive Statistics

	N	Mean	Std. Deviation
BMI	100	16.892	1.6766
Valid N (listwise)	100		

4.6.3 Descriptive Statistics

Since the population is normally distributed, select the mean and standard deviation to describe the characteristics of the sample.

1. Analyze → Descriptive Statistics → Descriptives.
2. In the Descriptives dialog box, enter *BMI* in the variable(s) list → select Options.
3. In the Descriptives: Options dialog box, select Mean and Standard Deviation → select Continue.
4. In the Descriptives dialog box, select OK.
5. SPSS Outcome (as shown in Fig. 4.8).

The mean BMI of 100 students aged 6 to 17 years is 16.892 kg/m^2, and the standard deviation is 1.6766 kg/m^2.

Chapter Summary
1. The most common continuous distribution is the normal distribution; the two parameters μ and σ completely define a normal curve.
2. Most commonly investigated characteristics of a set of data are the central tendency and variation. The measures of central tendency are arithmetic mean, geometric mean, and median; the measures of variation are range, interquartile range, variance, standard deviation, and coefficient of variance.

3. The partial regression coefficient could be influenced by dimensions, therefore, cannot be used to compare independent factors' impacts for dependent variable. Standardized partial regression coefficient eliminates the influence for different units; their absolute value could be used to compare their effects on the response variable.
4. For a normal distribution, use mean and standard deviation to describe the characteristics of a data set; for a skewed distribution, use median and interquartile range to describe the characteristics of a data set.

Chapter 5
Description of Categorical Variables

Dongliang He

Objectives
Relative measurement is often used to describe categorical variable. This
chapter introduces three kinds of frequently used relative measurements
including ratio, frequency, and intensity to explain why crude intensities cannot be directly compared with each other as well as to demonstrate how standardization approaches work.

Key Concepts
Ratio; Frequency; Intensity; Crude rate; Standardization

5.1 Introduction

A categorical variable, sometimes referred to a nominal variable, has two or more
categories without intrinsic order. For example, gender is a categorical variable with
two categories (male and female), but these two categories have no intrinsic order.
Hair color is another categorical variable with multiple categories (blonde, brown,
brunette, red, etc.) and also has no general consensus on their order. A categorical
variable is one that possesses categories without a clear order. If the categories of a
variable are clearly ordered, that variable would be an ordinal variable.

Categorical variables are often assigned as quantitative variables. For example,
gender may be assigned as 0 = male and 1 = female. Data are generally easy to
manipulate in an analysis spreadsheet when they are coded quantitatively.

D. He (✉)
School of Public Health, University of South China, Hengyang, China

© Zhengzhou University Press 2024   63
X. Guo, F. Xue (eds.), *Textbook of Medical Statistics*,
https://doi.org/10.1007/978-981-99-7390-3_5

Nevertheless, the variable remains categorical and is not truly measured as a number. In some cases, it is difficult to make a distinction.

To make comparisons among groups more meaningful, a rate may be used instead of raw numbers. A rate is defined as the number of cases of a particular outcome of interest that occurs and divided by the population size in a given time period. For example, we might be interested in the number of diagnosed ear infections for a specific group of elementary school students during a 2-month period.

5.2 Ratio, Frequency, and Intensity

In vital statistics and epidemiology, relative measures are widely used to describe the probability and intensity of certain events that may? the individuals in a population. These relative measures are often followed by the term "rate." In fact, there are three types of relative measures.

5.2.1 Ratio

A ratio is simply the proportion of any quantity to another, such as:

$$\text{Sex ratio of newly born babies} = \frac{\text{number of newly born girls}}{\text{number of newly born boys}} \tag{5.1}$$

and

$$\text{Body mass index} = \frac{\text{Weight}}{\text{Height}^2}\left(\text{kg/m}^2\right) \tag{5.2}$$

where the numerator and denominator may not necessarily have the same dimensions.

5.2.2 Relative Frequency

Relative frequency is a special type of ratio that both the numerator and denominator are counted numbers, with the numerator as a part of the denominator. When the denominator is large enough for a random sample, relative frequency approximately describes the chance of a certain event happening to the individuals in a population. For example, if 90 patients are cured among 100 treated ones, then

$$\text{Cure rate} = \frac{\text{number of cured}}{\text{number of treated}} = \frac{90}{100} \times 100\% = 90\% \tag{5.3}$$

There is no dimension for relative frequency, and the value is either a percentage or decimal within the interval of [0, 1].

5.2.3 Intensity

Intensity is another special type of ratio that the denominator is the total observed person-years during a certain period, and the numerator is the number of times a certain event occurred during that period. For example, the mortality rate is defined as

$$\text{Mortality rate of a certain year} = \frac{\text{Number of deaths during the year}}{\substack{\text{Person years exposed to the risk of death} \\ \text{during the year}}} \tag{5.4}$$

The dimension of the numerator is "persons" and that of the denominator is "persons × year." As a result, the dimension of the mortality rate is "persons/(persons × year)" or "1/year." If the denominator is regarded as the "adjusted total number of persons × 1 year," the mortality rate can be regarded as the adjusted relative frequency per year.

In general, intensity can be understood as the "relative frequency per unit of time," reflecting the chance of a certain event happening in a certain unit of time.

If an inference for a relative measure from a sample is needed, the type of relative measure must be recognized, whether it is simply a ratio or a relative frequency or intensity, due to the different statistical methods required for each separate type.

5.3 Crude Death Rate and Standardization

We will use the mortality rate as an example to show why primary intensities are not directly comparable and how standardization approaches work. Table 5.1 gives two sets of data for two cities, each of which includes the midyear population, the number of deaths during the year, and the mortality rate.

Judged from the primary data, the mortality rate seems to differ between the two cities. The mortality rate in City A is 11.1 per 1000 in the population, while the mortality rate in City B is 23.3 per 1000 in the population. Of these two groups, it appears that the risk of death in City B is higher than that in City A. Is this a valid conclusion?

Table 5.1 Data for the mortality rates of two cities

Cities	Midyear population ($\times 10^3$)	Number of deaths ($\times 10^3$)	Mortality rate (‰)
City A	5680	63	11.1
City B	5618	131	23.3
Total	11,298	194	17.2

Table 5.2 Data for age-specific mortality rates of two cities

	City A			City B		
Age group (year)	Midyear population ($\times 10^3$)	Number of deaths ($\times 10^3$)	Mortality rate (‰)	Midyear population ($\times 10^3$)	Number of deaths ($\times 10^3$)	Mortality rate (‰)
0~	400	2	5.0	288	1	3.5
15~	2000	10	5.0	238	1	4.2
30~	2000	15	7.5	794	5	6.3
45~	800	8	10.0	2000	18	9.0
60~	400	16	40.0	2000	70	35.0
75+	80	12	150.0	300	36	120.0
Total	5680	63	11.1	5618	131	23.3

A problem that often arises when primary rates for distinct groups are compared is that the populations may differ substantially with respect to important characteristics, such as age and sex. For example, if there are two populations from two different geographical areas, one composed entirely of males and the other entirely of females, it is difficult to determine whether a difference in their mortality rates is due to location or to gender. In this situation, gender is referred to as a *confounder*. Due to its association with both geographical area and death rate, it obscures the true relationship between the geographical area and the death.

To determine whether it is fair to describe that the risk of death in City B is higher than that in City A, the underlying structure of the two subpopulations should be compared, for the reason that age served as a *confounder*. Therefore, each group has been broken down according to age (see Table 5.2).

From the relative frequencies, it is clear that the two groups differ in age composition: there are more the elder in City B than in City A. The mortality rates of the subpopulations of City A are higher than those of the corresponding subpopulations of City B. Therefore, in order to make a more accurate comparison between the two cities, their respective age-specific mortality rates should be more carefully considered than the primary rates. Although the subgroup-specific rates provide a more accurate comparison among populations than the primary rates, there would be an overwhelming number of rates to compare in the condition that there are numerous subgroups. A comprehensive measure summarizing all subgroup-specific rates is often expected in applications, such as a comparison between different cities. Standardization helps summarize and adjust the imbalance of subgroup distributions by selecting a certain "standard" and calculating standardized rates.

5.3.1 Direct Method of Standardization

The direct method to adjust the differences among populations focuses on computing the overall rates that would result in, instead of having different distributions, all populations being compared have same standard composition. The first step is to select a "standard population." Then, the whole set of age-specific mortality rates would be applied to such a "standard population," and the "expected number of deaths" for each age group in the "standard population" would be calculated. Finally, the standardized mortality rate by the "standard population" would be calculated based on the total expected number of deaths.

Example 5.1 Using the population of City A in Table 5.2 as a "standard population," please compare the risk of death between the two cities under the direct standardization approach.

Solution: Column 2 of Table 5.2 refers to the standard population. Column 3 and 5 refer to the age-specific mortality rates of the two cities, respectively. Column 4 and 6 refer to the expected number of deaths for each age group if the mortality rates were applied to the "standard population." Dividing the total expected number of deaths by the total population of the "standard population" would result in the direct standardized mortality rates for the two cities (bottom cells of column 3 and 5, respectively). It can be concluded that the standardized mortality rate of City A is higher than that of City B. This is consistent with the conclusion obtained by the comparison of the corresponding age groups.

Note that the choice of a different standard age distribution—column 1 in Table 5.3—would lead to a different standardized mortality rate. Age-standardized mortality has no meaning by itself. It is just a construct that is calculated based on a hypothetical standard distribution. Unlike a primary or specific rate, it does not reflect the true mortality of City A or City B. Standardized mortality rates have meaning only when comparing two or more groups, although it has been shown that trends among the groups are generally unaffected by the choice of a standard population.

Table 5.3 The direct approach for standardized mortality rates of two cities

Age group (year) (1)	Standard population (10^3) (2)	City A		City B	
		Mortality rate (‰) (3)	Expected number of deaths (10^3) (4) = (2)*(3)	Mortality rate (‰) (5)	Expected number of deaths (10^3) (6) = (2)*(5)
0~	400	5.0	2.0	3.5	1.4
15~	2000	5.0	10.0	4.2	8.4
30~	2000	7.5	15.0	6.3	12.6
45~	800	10.0	8.0	9.0	7.2
60~	400	40.0	16.0	35.0	14.0
75+	80	150.0	12.0	120.0	9.6
Total	5680	11.1	63.0	9.4	53.2

5.3.2   Indirect Method of Standardization

Indirect standardization is different in both method and interpretation as opposed to the direct one. Instead of using the structure of the standard population, the specific rates are applied to the population under comparison, previously stratified by the variable to be controlled. The total number of expected cases is obtained this way. The standardized mortality ratio (SMR) is calculated by dividing the total number of observed cases by the total number of expected cases. This ratio allows a comparison of each population under study to the standard population. A conclusion can be reached by simply calculating and looking at the SMR. SMR higher than one (or 100% if expressed in percentages) indicates that the risk of death in the observed population is higher than what would be expected if it had the same experience or risk as the standard population. On the other hand, SMR lower than one (or 100%) indicates that the risk of death is lower in the observed population than expected if its distribution was the same as the reference population. The actual adjusted rates can also be calculated by the indirect method of multiplying the primary rate of every population by its SMR. Similar to using the direct method, a single value is obtained for every population. This value takes into account the compositional differences of the populations, even if it represents an artificial number.

Standardized mortality ratios are frequently used in epidemiology to compare different study groups, because they are easy to calculate and provide an estimate of the relative risk between the standard population and the population under study. However, it is inadequate when the rate ratios of the groups under study and the population of reference are not homogeneous in the different strata. The SMRs of different causes in a population may also be calculated on a single standard.

Example 5.2 In 1999, the primary mortality rate in Colombia was 4.4 per 1000, with variations between 1.8 per 1000 in the population in the district of Vichada and 6.9 per 1000 in the population in Quindío. There may be possible significant differences in the observed mortality (or in the risk of death) in the country and its districts. The case of the state of Vichada is presented in this example. Please use the indirect standardization method to compare the mortality in Vichada with the mortality in Colombia in general in 1999.

Solution: In order to use the indirect method, the following pieces of information are needed: (1) the age-specific mortality rates by age group in Colombia; (2) the population of the state of Vichada stratified by age; and (3) the total number of deaths observed in Vichada. The first step is to calculate the expected number of deaths in Vichada by applying the standard rates to the population (column 5 = (2) × (3)). The expected deaths are summed up, and SMR is calculated by dividing the total number of observed deaths through the expected deaths in Vichada (Table 5.4).

$$\text{SMR for Vichada} = \frac{142}{267} \times 100\% = 53\%$$

$$(5.5)$$

Table 5.4 The indirect approach for standardized mortality rates of Vichada

Age distribution (1)	Mortality rate in Colombia, 1999 (10^{-5}) (2)	Population in Vichada (3)	Number of deaths observed (4)	Number of deaths expected (5)
0–4	339	11,392	61	39
5–14	34	21,930	5	7
15–44	219	38,244	27	84
45–64	752	7083	22	53
65 +	4573	1839	27	84
		80,488	142	267

The SMR of 53% indicates that in the population of Vichada, the risk of death is 47% less than expected according to the mortality standards of all of Colombia when controlling for the age.

5.3.3 The Use of Standardized Rates

Standardized rates are encountered frequently in the study of vital statistics. However, with any summary measure, adjusted rates may present great differences between groups, which may be important for explaining changes in the rates due to or associated with the variable that is adjusted for. If there are no confounding factors such as age or gender, and if comparisons between groups are not required, primary rates are generally sufficient. Standardized rates (a single number summary of the situation in each population being considered) should be used only if one or more confounders are present and a comparison is desired.

In practice, the direct method of standardization is used much more frequently than the indirect method. However, the direct method requires that subgroup-specific rates are available for all population being compared. If subgroup-specific rates are not available, the indirect method should be used instead. Furthermore, when the subgroup-specific rates are available but calculated based on very small numbers, the indirect method is still preferred. The selection of standard population or standard mortality rates is equally important. There are usually three alternatives: the population or mortality rates of the world, a country, or a province may be used; the pool of the two populations or the pooled estimation of the age-specific mortality rates may be used; and a population or the estimation of the age-specific mortality rates may be used. Please note that the standardization rates would change, depending on the choice of a standard population or standard mortality rates.

In short, adjusted rates allow for more exact comparisons between populations. This is important, because it can be used to set disease control priorities among the groups. Nevertheless, primary rates are the only indicators of the real dimension or magnitude of a problem, thus remaining a valuable public health measurement.

Chapter Summary

1. Each of the three types of relative measures, ratio, frequency, and intensity, has its specific meaning and purpose.
2. Primary mortalities or intensities are not directly comparable when subpopulations have different underlying structures. In these scenarios, the standardization approaches should be chosen.
3. The direct method of adjusting for differences among populations focuses on computing the overall rates that all populations being compared would have if they have the same standard composition. Indirect standardization uses its specific rates and applies them to the populations under comparison.

Chapter 6
Inferential Statistics: Confidence Interval

Ya Fang and Ying Hu

There are mainly two major tasks for statistical work to accomplish. One is statistical description and the other is statistical inference. Inferential statistics uses sample information to infer population information. Inferential statistics includes confidence interval estimation and hypothesis test. Confidence interval estimation is a process to calculate with sample statistics and get an interval based on certain probability which includes population parameter. Details will be discussed in this chapter.

Objectives
A confidence interval gives an estimated range of values which is with certain probability to include an unknown population parameter. The estimated range is calculated from a given set of sample data. The objective of this chapter is to give a detailed description of the basic concept and calculations of confidence intervals of a population mean or proportion.

Key Concepts
Sampling error; *t*-Distribution; Confidence interval

Y. Fang (✉)
School of Public Health of Xiamen University, Xiamen, China
e-mail: fangya@xmu.edu.cn

Y. Hu
School of Health Science of Wuhan University, Wuhan, China

© Zhengzhou University Press 2024
X. Guo, F. Xue (eds.), *Textbook of Medical Statistics*,
https://doi.org/10.1007/978-981-99-7390-3_6

6.1   Introduction

The preceding chapter discusses normal distributions. Assuming the sample mean and standard deviation of a sample from a population are found, estimates of the equivalent population parameters can be obtained from this sample. $\bar{X}$ and S are the sample estimates of population μ and σ, respectively. However, how accurate are these estimates? Obviously, a sample does not include the entire population. Investigators usually expect to indicate the variabilities that exist among the estimates of different samples. To indicate this variability, they use interval estimates. The process of drawing conclusions about an entire population based on the information in a sample is defined as statistical inference.

6.2   *t*-Distribution and Binomial Distribution

6.2.1   *Sampling Distribution and Standard Error*

Assume that researchers are interested in the true value of a population mean, μ. In fact, the value of μ is unknown before we go through the whole population, but the knowledge about μ can be obtained from sample data. Nevertheless, there is a possibility of not reaching the true value of the parameter, because statistical inference is usually based on certain level of accuracy. In addition, different samples drawn from the same population could have different values of the sample statistic.

Sampling errors are those which occur due to the nature of sampling. The sample selected from the population is one of all possible samples. Any value calculated from the sample data is called the sample statistic. Due to the fact that only a certain part of the population is represented in the sample, the sample statistic may or may not be close estimate to the population parameter. If the statistic is $\bar{X}$ and the true value of the corresponding population parameter is μ, the difference, $\bar{X} - \mu$, is called the sampling error that must be taken into account in the statistical reference. It is essential to note that a statistic is a variable that may be with sampling error when the population parameter is unknown. Therefore, it is important to estimate the standard error from the sample.

Since the observations are usually requested to be collected from a random sample, statistical theory provides a probabilistic estimation of the sampling error for this particular sample. The sampling error of sample means often expressed in terms of the standard error. In statistics, a sampling distribution is the distribution of a given statistic based on random sampling of sample size n. It is considered to be the distribution of the statistic for all possible samples with a given size from a specific population.

The sampling distribution depends on the underlying distribution of the population, the statistic being considered, and the sample size used. For example, consider a normal population with mean μ and variance σ^2. Assume that samples of a given size from this population are repeatedly taken, and the average value for each sample is calculated. Each sample has its own average value, and the distribution of these averages is so called the "sampling distribution of the sample mean." This distribution is normal if the underlying population distribution is normal. Under circumstance, when central limit theorem could be applied, even the population is not normal, the sampling distribution still could be normal.

The standard deviation of different sample means (sampling distribution) is referred to as the standard error. The standard error is calculated by:

$$\sigma_{\bar{x}} = \frac{\sigma}{\sqrt{n}} \tag{6.1}$$

where σ is the standard deviation of the population distribution and n is the number of subjects in the sample. The standard error can generally be reduced by increasing the sample size and by improving the sampling design (i.e., decreasing standard variation).

In practical applications, the true value of the population's standard deviation is usually unknown. Instead, the sample standard deviation is used to calculate standard error:

$$S_{\bar{x}} = \frac{S}{\sqrt{n}} \tag{6.2}$$

Example 6.1 Among the adults in District X, the distribution of the red-cell count is roughly normal distribution. A total of 144 subjects are randomly selected from this population. The mean of the red-cell count of the sample is 5.38 (10^{12}/L), and the standard deviation is 0.42 (10^{12}/L). What would be the standard error?

Solution: According to Formula (6.2), the standard error would be: $S_{\bar{x}} = \dfrac{s}{\sqrt{n}} = \dfrac{0.42}{\sqrt{144}} = \dfrac{0.42}{12} = 0.035.$

6.2.2 t-Distribution

If X is a variable which complies with normal distribution, that is $X - N(\mu, \sigma^2)$, the sample mean $\bar{X}$, of n-subjects from the sample, is also normally distributed with mean $\bar{X}$ and variance $\sigma_{\bar{x}}^2$.

$$\bar{X} - N\left(\mu, \sigma_{\bar{x}}^2\right)$$

The standardized variable:

$$u = \frac{\bar{X} - \mu}{\sigma / \sqrt{n}} = \frac{\bar{X} - \mu}{\sigma_{\bar{x}}} \tag{6.3}$$

is the difference of the sample mean from the population mean divided by standard error. When using normal distribution to deal with parameter estimation problems, there are many distribution lines for normal distribution with different mean and standard error. In order to simplify the process, standard normal distribution is applied. Normal distribution is standardized by its own distribution's standard deviation as a "unit length." The U-distribution is symmetric, with a mean of 0 and a standard deviation of 1:

$$u - N(0,1)$$

Therefore, if the variance, σ^2, of a normal distribution is known, the sample mean is transformed into a standard normal variable. If the variance, σ^2, is unknown, replace σ^2 with the sample variance, S^2. Then the distribution curve depends on the sample size, which is shown in the t-distribution curve that is influenced by degree of freedom-v. Degree of freedom is a parameter of the t-distribution. Fortunately, when the sample size is large enough, t-distribution is approaching standard normal distribution.

The above v-dependent distribution is regarded as a "Student's t-distribution," or simply, "t-distribution." The distribution of t (for n-observation samples) with $(n - 1)$ degrees of freedom (df or denoted by the Greek letter "v") is denoted as t_{n-1}.

$$t = \frac{\overline{X} - \mu}{S / \sqrt{n}}, \quad v = n - 1 \tag{6.4}$$

The t-distribution curve is symmetric and bell-shaped, similar to a normal distribution. Because the t-distribution has a larger standard deviation than u-distribution, it is also with wider and higher tails. Thus, with the same percentage of confidence interval, the estimation of population parameter is wider for t-distribution than u-distribution. As the sample size increases, the value of df also increases. The t-distribution becomes almost the same as the standard normal distribution, so either t or u can be used when sample size is large enough (Fig. 6.1).

In probability and statistics, the t-distribution is a continuous probability distribution that is used when estimating mean of a normally distributed population in

Fig. 6.1 A standard normal (u) distribution and t-distributions with $v = 1$ and 5

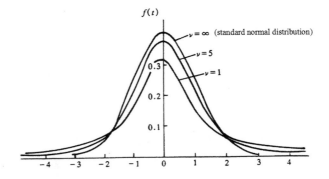

situations where the sample size is small and population standard deviation is unknown. It is used in a number of statistical analyses, including the construction of confidence intervals for the corresponding population mean according to the sample information. A student's t-test could be used for assessing the statistical significance of the difference between means from a sample and a population, two samples, or paired samples.

When the t-distribution is used to answer statistical questions, the area under the curve should be calculated, in which it is similar to using a u-distribution. The area can be computed by using calculus to integrate a mathematical function. However, a t-distribution table lists selected values for t-distributions with ν degrees of freedom for a range of one-sided or two-sided critical regions. The table of t-Distribution in the Appendix gives the critical values for the t-distributions corresponding to areas in the tail of the distribution equal to 0.10, 0.05, 0.02, 0.01, and 0.001, for both two-tailed and one-tailed tests. For example, take the corresponding degree of freedom, which is usually indicated as v, and find the corresponding probability. Carefully choose the one-sided or two-sided value. For example, check out five as degrees of freedom and 0.05 for a two-sided (0.025 for one-sided) test. The value of that entry is "2.571." The sum of the area under the curve from $-\infty$ to -2.571 and from 2.571 to $+\infty$ is 0.05, which implies that Pr $(-2.571 < t < 2.571) = 0.95$. The area under the curve from 2.571 to $+\infty$ is 0.025, which means that Pr $(-\infty < t \leq 2.571) = 0.975$. Pr $(t > 2.571)$ can be calculated by the symmetry of the distribution,

$$\Pr(t > 2.571) = 1 - \Pr(t \leq 2.571) = 1 - 0.975 = 0.025$$

When looking at the table of critical values, the following should be notified. (1) The probabilities for a two-tailed distribution are exactly twice of those for a one-tailed distribution for the same t-value. For example, 2.447 standard deviations from the mean correspond to a 5% two-tailed critical value with 6 degrees of freedom, or a corresponding 2.5% one-tailed critical value. (2) For identical probabilities, the value decreases with increasing degrees of freedom. (3) For identical degrees of freedom, the probability decreases with increasing values. (4) When $\nu \to +\infty$, the t value is just the u value for the corresponding probability.

It must be assumed that the observations comply with t-distribution when using a t-distribution. When the observations don't comply with t-distribution, another appropriate method should be considered.

6.2.3   Binomial Distribution

In many cases, data arises in the form of counts, which are summarized by the number of observations in the group that represents one of the two outcomes (e.g., success or failure, yes or no, and positive or negative). Assume an event has only binary outcomes, denoted as A and B. The probability of A is denoted by π or $P(A) = \pi$.

The probability of B must therefore be $1 - \pi$, because B occurs if A does not. If an experiment involving this event is repeated n times, and the outcomes are independent of one another, what is the probability of outcome A occurring exactly X times? A binomial distribution is used to provide the probability of observing X successes in n trials, with the probability of success on a single trial denoted by p.

The binomial distribution describes the behavior of a count variable X if the following conditions apply. (1) The number of observations, n, is fixed. (2) Each observation is independent. (3) Each observation represents one of the two mutually exclusive outcomes. (4) The probability of "success," π, is the same for each outcome.

The following formula gives the probability of observing exactly X successes:

$$P(X) = \binom{n}{X} \pi^X (1-\pi)^{n-X} \tag{6.5}$$

In case of $X - B(n, \pi)$, the binomial mean of X, or the expected number of successes in n trials, is $E(X) = n\pi$. The standard deviation is $\sigma = \sqrt{n\pi(1-\pi)}$. The standard deviation is a measure of dispersion tendency, increasing with n and decreasing as π approaches either 0 or 1.

Studies involving dichotomous variables often use a proportion instead of a number to present data. This proportion is calculated by dividing X by n. The mean of the proportion (μ_p) becomes π, and the standard deviation becomes:

$$\sigma_p = \sqrt{\frac{\pi(1-\pi)}{n}} \tag{6.6}$$

When the population proportion is unknown, the sample proportion is used to estimate π. The estimation of σ_p is:

$$S_p = \sqrt{\frac{p(1-p)}{n}} \tag{6.7}$$

For example, with $X - B(20, 0.3)$, the probability of observing exactly five successes is:

$$P(5) = \binom{20}{5} 0.3^5 (1-0.3)^{15} = 0.1789$$

The mean and variance are:

$$\mu = 20 \times 0.3 = 6, \ Var(X) = 20 \times 0.3 \times 0.7 = 4.2$$

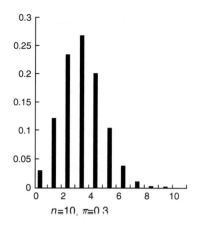
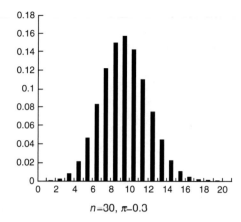

Fig. 6.2 Binomial distributions

The binomial distribution is a discrete probability distribution that is symmetric when p is equal to or close to 0.5. Even p is not equal to 0.5, but the number of trials (n) is large, the binomial distribution is approximately equal to the normal distribution (Fig. 6.2). Usually, when $n\pi$ and $n(1 - \pi) > 5$ standards exist, the binomial distribution could be considered as approximating the normal distribution.

6.3   Central Limit Theorem

The properties of the sampling distribution are the basis for one of the most important theorems in statistics—the central limit theorem.

Let X be a continuous random variable described by a probability density function with mean μ and variance σ^2. The sampling distribution of the mean based on repeated random samples of size n has the following properties:

1. The mean of the sampling distribution, or the mean of the means, is equal to the population mean μ based on the individual observations.
2. The standard deviation for the sampling distribution of the mean is $\sigma / \sqrt{n}$, which is called the standard error (SE) of the mean.
3. If the distribution of the population is normal, the sampling distribution of the mean is also normal. Most importantly, the variable is from a random sample of size n, that is, a series of independent and normally distributed random variables drawn from distributions of expected values given by μ and variance given by σ^2. For large enough sample size, the sampling distribution of the mean is approximately normally distributed, regardless of the shape of the original population distribution.

6.4   Confidence Interval

6.4.1   Confidence Interval for a Mean

Usually, the large population mean and standard deviation are unknown. Our goal is to estimate these unknown parameters. The standard way is to use the sample mean and standard deviation as a best estimate of the true population mean and standard deviation. We consider that "best estimate" as a point estimate. For example, $\bar{X}$ is a point estimate for μ, and S is a point estimate for σ.

However, the true population mean or standard deviation may be larger or smaller than the sample mean or standard deviation. The central limit theorem states that if many samples are taken, the means of all the samples will vary within an interval around the population mean. Instead of a point estimate, the interval around $\bar{X}$ (such that there is with assumed probability that the true population mean falls into this interval) is the estimate of interest. This interval is called a confidence interval (*CI*), and the probability is called the confidence level $(1 - \alpha)$. The boundaries of a confidence interval are determined by the confidence level, which is usually set at 95% to comply with the 5% convention of statistical significance in hypothesis testing. In some cases, 90% or 99% confidence intervals are required. Confidence intervals are composed of a lower confidence limit (C_L) and upper confidence limit (C_U).

There are two methods of calculating a confidence interval:

1. Confidence interval for a mean when the population standard deviation is unknown:

When the population is normal, but the sample size is not large enough, use a t-distribution. The distribution has $n - 1$ degrees of freedom.

$$P\left(-t_{\alpha/2,\upsilon} < \frac{\bar{X} - \mu}{S_{\bar{X}}} < t_{\alpha/2,\upsilon}\right) = 1 - \alpha$$

The two-sided $(1 - \alpha)$ confidence interval of a population mean is:

$$\bar{X} - t_{\alpha/2,\upsilon} S_{\bar{X}} < \mu < \bar{X} + t_{\alpha/2,\upsilon} S_{\bar{X}}$$

It can also be expressed as

$$\left(\bar{X} - t_{\alpha/2,\upsilon} S_{\bar{X}}, \ \bar{X} + t_{\alpha/2,\upsilon} S_{\bar{X}}\right) \quad \text{or} \quad \bar{X} \pm t_{\alpha/2,\upsilon} S_{\bar{X}} \tag{6.8}$$

The one-sided $(1 - \alpha)$ confidence interval of a population mean is:

$$\mu > \bar{X} - t_{\alpha,\upsilon} S_{\bar{X}} \quad \text{or} \quad \mu < \bar{X} + t_{\alpha,\upsilon} S_{\bar{X}} \tag{6.9}$$

Example 6.2 The values of fasting plasma glucose in healthy adults approximately follow a normal distribution. A random sample of 25 healthy adults is selected from this population. The sample mean of the fasting plasma glucose is 4.91 mmol/L, and the standard deviation is 0.72 mmol/L. What would be the 95% confidence interval of the population mean of the fasting plasma glucose in healthy adults?

Solution: According to Formula (6.8),

$$C_\mathrm{L} = \bar{X} - t_{\alpha/2,\upsilon} \cdot S_{\bar{X}} = 4.91 - 2.064 \times 0.72 / \sqrt{25} = 4.613 \ (\mathrm{mmol}/\mathrm{L}),$$

$$C_\mathrm{U} = \bar{X} + t_{\alpha/2,\upsilon} \cdot S_{\bar{X}} = 4.91 + 2.064 \times 0.72 / \sqrt{25} = 5.207 \ (\mathrm{mmol}/\mathrm{L}).$$

The 95% confidence interval would be (4.613, 5.207) mmol/L.

2. Confidence interval for a mean when the σ is known or the σ is not known, and sample size is large enough.

According to the principle of normal distributions, the confidence interval can be calculated based on the following:
When σ is known,

$$\left(\bar{X} - u_{\alpha/2} \times \sigma_{\bar{X}}, \quad \bar{X} + u_{\alpha/2} \times \sigma_{\bar{X}} \right) \tag{6.10}$$

When σ is not known and the sample size is large enough ($n > 100$),

$$\left(\bar{X} - u_{\alpha/2} \times S_{\bar{X}}, \quad \bar{X} + u_{\alpha/2} \times S_{\bar{X}} \right) \tag{6.11}$$

Example 6.3 For Example 6.1, a total of 144 subjects, the mean of the red-cell count of the sample is 5.38 (10^{12}/L), and the standard deviation is 0.42 (10^{12}/L). What would be the 95% confidence interval of the red-cell count among adults in District X?

Solution: According to Formula (6.11), the 95% confidence interval would be:

$$\left(5.38 - 1.96 \times 0.035, \quad 5.38 + 1.96 \times 0.035 \right) \quad \text{or} \quad \left(5.31, 5.45 \right) \times 10^{12} / \mathrm{L}.$$

6.4.2 Confidence Interval for a Proportion

The central limit theorem also applies to a binomial distribution, when $n\pi$ and $n(1 - \pi) > 5$. However, for very extreme probabilities, a sample size of 30 or more may still be inadequate under the sample proportion close to zero or one. The 95% confidence intervals for the true population proportion π are given by

$$p \pm u_{\alpha/2} \cdot S_p \tag{6.12}$$

Example 6.4 A random sample of 110 children with pneumonia is injected with azithromycin, among which 50 children are cured. What would be the 95% confidence interval for the true proportion of the cure rate?

Solution: The cure rate of the sample is $P = 50/110 = 0.454$,

According to Formula (6.7),

$$S_p = \sqrt{\frac{0.454(1-0.454)}{110}} = 0.0475$$

According to Formula (6.11), the 95% confidence interval would be:

$$(0.454 - 1.96 \times 0.0475, \quad 0.454 + 1.96 \times 0.0475) \quad \text{or} \quad (0.361, 0.547).$$

Chapter Summary
1. In statistics, a sampling distribution is the distribution of the statistic for all possible samples with a given size from the same population. The sampling distribution depends on the underlying distribution of the population. The standard error is an estimation of the standard deviation of the sampling distribution.
2. The student's t-distribution is symmetric and bell-shaped like a normal distribution. Because the t-distribution has a larger standard deviation, it is lower, wider, and its tails are higher than those for the u-distribution. As the sample size increases, the t-distribution approaches the standard normal distribution. The binomial distribution is a discrete probability distribution under $np > 5$ and $n(1 - p) > 5$, the binomial distribution is approximately equal to the normal distribution.
3. A confidence interval, calculated from a given set of sample data, gives an estimated range of values which includes an unknown population parameter to the probability extent. The boundaries of a confidence interval are determined by the confidence level which is usually set at 95% to comply with the 5% convention of statistical significance in hypothesis testing.

Chapter 7
Inferential Statistics: *t*-Tests

Qi Gao and Suling Zhu

Objectives
Hypothesis testing permits investigators to generalize study results from a sample to the population. This chapter introduces this statistical procedure and the analysis of the difference between two treatments using the *t*-test for significance. Also, it discusses when, why, and how to appropriately perform a *t*-test and present the results. Three types of *t*-tests will be discussed in this chapter, as well as the conditions under which each of these types is appropriate. Examples are given to demonstrate the procedures of these three types of *t*-tests using SPSS software.

Key Concepts
Hypothesis testing; One-sample *t*-test; Two-sample *t*-test; Paired-sample *t*-test; Equal variances; Type I error; Type II error; Power

7.1 Introduction

When comparing two treatments or characters, relying on only the numerical differences is inadequate. Since each group is represented by only a sample of observations, the numerical values would be changed with the different possible samples.

Q. Gao (✉)
School of Public Health, Capital Medical University, Beijing, China
e-mail: gaoqi@ccmu.edu.cn

S. Zhu
School of Public Health, Lanzhou University, Lanzhou, China

© Zhengzhou University Press 2024
X. Guo, F. Xue (eds.), *Textbook of Medical Statistics*,
https://doi.org/10.1007/978-981-99-7390-3_7

81

Statistical science provides an objective procedure, called a test of significance, to distinguish whether the observed difference suggests any real difference between the two groups or if the difference is due to chance.

A statistical hypothesis test is a method of making decisions using data from either a controlled experiment or an observational study. In statistics, a result is considered to be statistically significant if it is unlikely to have occurred by chance alone, according to a predetermined threshold probability (i.e., the significance level). The general steps of hypothesis testing are as follows.

Make an assumption that there is no difference (technically known as the null hypothesis). The test of significance is designed to assess the strength of the evidence against the null hypothesis. Usually, the null hypothesis is a statement of "no effect" or "no difference." This is often abbreviated as H_0. The statement that is suspected to be true, as opposed to the null hypothesis, is known as the alternate hypothesis and is abbreviated as H_1.

Find a suitable estimate (technically known as the test statistic). Each specific survey or experiment has a different test statistic, but these statistics are usually constructed based on the two principles—the statistic estimates the parameter and measures the distance of the estimate from the hypothesized value.

Find the probability of observing a specific value of the test statistic or more extreme values (technically known as the P-value), assuming that the null hypothesis is true. As the P-value gets smaller, the evidence against the null hypothesis grows stronger.

Make a decision to either reject the null hypothesis or fail to reject the null hypothesis. Notice that the null hypothesis has not been proven to be true or false, and all that has been achieved is to show that the observed data are either not unusual (if the P-value is large) or highly unusual (if the P-value is small). How small must the P-value be to reject the null hypothesis? The decisive value of the P-value is known as the significance level and is denoted by the Greek letter α.

7.2 Hypothesis Testing

Setting up testing hypotheses is an essential part of statistical inferences. In order to formulate such a test, there must be a theory that has been proposed. The theory is either believed to be true or is only used as a basis for an argument but has not been proved. For example, claiming that a new drug is better than the current drug for treatment of the same symptoms is one possible proposal.

In each problem considered, the question of interest can be simplified into two competing hypotheses—the null hypothesis (denoted *as* H_0) and the alternative hypothesis (denoted as H_1). Note that these two competing claims are not treated on an equal basis—special consideration is given to the null hypothesis. There are two common situations:

1. The experiment has been carried out in an attempt to disprove or reject a particular hypothesis (i.e., the null hypothesis). Thus, the null hypothesis is given priority, so it cannot be rejected unless there is sufficient strong evidence against it. For example,

   H_0: There is no difference between a new drug and the current drug for treatment of the same symptoms.

   H_1: There is a difference between the new and current drugs.

2. If one of the two hypotheses is "simpler," then that hypothesis is given priority, so that a more "complicated" theory is not adopted unless there is sufficient evidence against the "simpler one." For example, it is "simpler" to claim that there is no difference between a new drug and the current drug for treatment of the same symptoms than it is to declare that there is a difference.

The hypotheses are often statements about population parameters, such as expected values and variance. For instance, H_0 might state that the expected value of the height of 10-year old boys is not different from that of 10-year old girls in the Chinese population. A hypothesis could also be a statement about the distributional form of a characteristic of interest, such as whether the height of 10-year old boys is normally distributed within the Chinese population.

The outcome of a hypothesis test is either "reject H_0 in favor of H_1" or "fail to reject H_0."

7.2.1 Null Hypothesis and Alternative Hypothesis

The null hypothesis, H_0, represents a proposed theory, either because it is believed to be true or because it is the basis for an argument but has not been proved. For example, the null hypothesis in a clinical trial of a new drug might be that the new drug is no better, on average, than the current drug. The null hypothesis would be written as:

H_0: There is no difference between the two drugs on average.

The null hypothesis is given special consideration, because it relates to the statement being tested, whereas the alternative hypothesis relates to the statement to be accepted if the null hypothesis is rejected.

The alternative hypothesis, H_1, is a statement of what a statistical hypothesis test is set up to establish. For example, the alternative hypothesis in a clinical trial of a new drug might be that the new drug has a different effect compared to that of the current drug. The alternative hypothesis would be written as:

H_1: The two drugs have different effects on average.

The alternative hypothesis could also be that the new drug is better, on average, than the current drug. In this case, it would be written as:

H_1: The new drug is better than the current drug on average.

The final conclusion once the test has been carried out is always given in terms of the null hypothesis. The conclusion is either "reject H_0 in favor of H_1" or "fail to reject H_0"; the conclusion is *never* stated as either "reject H_1" or "accept H_1."

If the conclusion is "fail to reject H_0," it does not necessarily mean that the null hypothesis is true—it only suggests that there is not sufficient evidence against H_0 in favor of H_1. On the other hand, rejecting the null hypothesis suggests that the alternative hypothesis *may* be true.

7.2.2 Test Statistic

A test statistic is a quantity calculated from sample data. Its value is used to determine whether or not the null hypothesis should be rejected in the hypothesis test. The choice of the test statistic depends on the presumed probability model and the hypothesis under questions.

7.2.3 P-Values

The probability value (*P*-value) of a statistical hypothesis test is the probability of getting a value of the test statistic as extreme as or more extreme than that observed by chance alone, if the null hypothesis (H_0) is true. It is the probability of incorrectly rejecting the null hypothesis if it is in fact true and equal to the significance level of the test for which the null hypothesis can be rejected. The *P*-value is the actual significance level of the test, and the result is statistically significant if *P*-value is smaller than significance level α. If the null hypothesis is rejected at the 5% significance level, it would be reported as $P < 0.05$.

Small *P*-values suggest that the null hypothesis is unlikely to be true. The smaller that the *P*-value is, the more convincing is the rejection of the null hypothesis. *P*-values indicate the strength of the evidence for rejecting the null hypothesis H_0 rather than the simple conclusion of "reject H_0" or "fail to reject H_0."

7.2.4 One-Sided Test and Two-Sided Test

A one-sided test (also referred to as a one-tailed test) of significance is a statistical hypothesis test in which the values for which the null hypothesis can be rejected are located entirely in one tail of the probability distribution. In other words, the critical region for a one-sided test is the set of values less than or greater than the critical value of the test.

A two-sided test is a statistical hypothesis test in which the values for which the null hypothesis, H_0, can be rejected are located in both tails of the probability distribution. A two-sided test is also referred to as a two-tailed test of significance.

The choice between a one-sided and a two-sided test is determined by the purpose of the investigation. For example, suppose a manufacturer's claim that there is an average of 50 matches in a box is tested. The following hypotheses would be set up as:

$$H_0 : \mu = 50$$

against H_1: $\mu < 50$ or H_1: $\mu > 50$.

Either of the two alternative hypotheses would lead to a one-sided test. Presumably, the null hypothesis would be tested against the first alternative hypothesis, since it would be more useful to know if there is likely to be less than 50 matches on average in a box (no one would complain if they got the correct number or more than the correct number of matches in a box).

In this case, nothing specific can be said about the average number of matches in a box. The only conclusion if the null hypothesis is rejected would be that the average number of matches in a box is likely to be less than or greater than 50.

7.3   One-Sample *t*-Test

A one-sample *t*-test is used for comparing sample mean with a known value. Specifically, a single sample is collected, and the corresponding sample mean is compared to a value of interest that is not based on the current sample. The purpose of the one-sample *t*-test is to determine whether there is sufficient evidence to conclude that the mean of the population from which the sample is taken is different from the specified value.

When performing a one-sample *t*-test, there may be a preconceived assumption about the direction of the findings; a one- or two-tailed test may be used depending on the design of the study.

If the population mean differs from the hypothesized value in a direction of interest, a one-tailed test would be used. For example, the purpose is to reject the null hypothesis only if there is sufficient evidence that the mean is larger than the value hypothesized in the null hypothesis (i.e., μ_0), the hypotheses are as follows:

H_0: $\mu = \mu_0$ (the population mean is equal to the hypothesized value μ_0)
H_1: $\mu > \mu_0$ (the population mean is greater than μ_0)

In the basic hypotheses for a two-tailed test, μ denotes the mean of the population from which the sample was selected, and μ_0 denotes the hypothesized value of this mean. The hypotheses are as follows:

H_0: $\mu = \mu_0$ (the population mean is equal to the hypothesized value μ_0)
H_1: $\mu \neq \mu_0$ (the population mean is not equal to μ_0)

7.3.1   Assumptions of a One-Sample t-Test

The assumptions for a one-sample t-test conclude: (1) dependent variables should be normally distributed; (2) samples drawn from the population should be random; (3) subjects of the samples should be independent; and (4) the preset population mean should be known.

7.3.2   Procedure for a One-Sample t-Test

Testing for the difference between a sample mean and a known value proceeds as follows:

1. State the null hypothesis and alternative hypothesis, and specify the level of significance.

   (a) Set up null hypothesis: In a one-sample t-test, the null hypothesis assumes that there is no significant difference between the population mean which the sample man represents and the known population mean.
   (b) Alternative hypothesis: In a one-sample t-test, the alternative hypothesis assumes that there is a significant difference between the population mean and the known population mean.
   (c) Specify the level of significance, and determine the critical values.

2. Calculate the statistic of the one-sample t-test by using the following formula

$$t = \frac{\bar{X} - \mu_0}{S / \sqrt{n}} \tag{7.1}$$

where t is t-test statistic, $\bar{X}$ is sample mean, μ_0 is known population mean, n is sample size, S is standard deviation that can be calculated as following formula

$$S = \sqrt{\frac{\sum \left(X - \bar{X} \right)^2}{n-1}} \tag{7.2}$$

   The degrees of freedom is $\nu = n - 1$.
3. Reach a conclusion, and interpret the result: In a one-sample t-test, decide whether or not the sample mean and the population mean are different. In hypothesis testing, the statistic t is compared with critical values in the statistical table (Appendix: Table of t distribution). If the calculated statistic is equal to or greater than the critical value, then reject the null hypothesis; otherwise, fail to reject the null hypothesis.

Example 7.1 According to a large number of surveys, the pulse of healthy adult males is 72 times/min, and standard deviation σ in the normal population was unknown. Based on a random sample of $n = 36$ healthy adult males in a mountainous area with a sample mean is $=75.9167$ times/min and sample standard deviation $S = 1.8574$ times/min, the sample data are listed in Table 7.1. Is it likely that the sample came from a population with a mean $\mu = 72$ times/min or from a population with a mean $\mu \neq 72$ times/min?

To test the hypothesis that the mean pulse of healthy adult males in the mountainous area is equal to that of the normal population, proceed as follows:

1. State the appropriate null and alternative hypotheses.

    The null hypothesis H_0: $\mu_{mountainous} = \mu_0 = \mu_{normal} = 72$ times/min. This means that mean pulse of healthy adult males in the mountainous area population is at most that of the normal population.

    The alternative hypothesis H_1: $\mu_{mountainous} \neq \mu_0 = \mu_{normal} = 72$ times/min.
2. Specify the level of significance.

    Suppose that $\alpha = 0.05$ and a two-tailed test.
3. Determine the appropriate technique. Since σ is unknown, a *t*-test is used.
4. Determine the critical values.

    For $\alpha = 0.05$, the critical t value is $t_{0.05/2, n-1} = t_{0.05/2,35} = 2.030$.
5. Collect the data and compute the test statistic.

    Suppose the sample results are $n = 36$, $\overline{X} = 75.9167$ times/min. From the Formula 7.1,

$$t = \frac{\overline{X} - \mu_0}{S/\sqrt{n}} = \frac{75.9167 - 72}{1.85742/\sqrt{36}} = 12.6521$$

6. Reach a conclusion and interpret the result.

    Since $t = 12.6521 > t_{0.05/2,35} = 2.030$, reject the null hypothesis, and conclude that healthy adult males in the mountainous area have *significantly higher* pulse levels on average than the normal healthy adult males.

Table 7.1 Pulse of healthy adult males in a mountainous area

Number	Pulse	Number	Pulse	Number	Pulse
1	75.00	13	77.00	25	76.00
2	77.00	14	74.00	26	78.00
3	76.00	15	77.00	27	76.00
4	73.00	16	80.00	28	76.00
5	75.00	17	76.00	29	77.00
6	73.00	18	74.00	30	76.00
7	79.00	19	75.00	31	75.00
8	78.00	20	76.00	32	78.00
9	76.00	21	74.00	33	75.00
10	73.00	22	78.00	34	77.00
11	72.00	23	74.00	35	76.00
12	79.00	24	77.00	36	75.00

7.4 Paired-Sample t-Test

Example 7.2 30 volunteer participants were given a diet pill, and their weights (kg) were measured before and after 2 months, respectively, and the weights losses data are listed in Table 7.2. Please try to determine whether the pill is effective for losing weight.

In this study, each participant accounts for a pair of observations, so there are two issues to consider:

1. The two sets of measurements are not independent, since they were taken from the same participant, and each participant served as his own "control." Thus, this design accounts for individual (biological) participant variability.
2. It is not appropriate to think that there are $2n$ distinct (independent) data points (or units of information) available, since each data point on the same subject provides a great deal of information on the subsequent data points collected on the same subject.

In a random sample of size n paired observations, compute the sample mean of the differences between the pairs of observations ($di = x_{Ci} - x_{Ti}, i = 1, ..., n$), where "C" means control and "T" means treatment. Carry out the test like a usual single-sample t-test based on these differences.

1. State the null hypothesis.

   H_0: $\delta = 0$, where δ is the difference mean between the control and treatment.
2. Set up the alternative hypothesis.

   (a) One-sided test: H_1: $\delta < 0$ or H_1: $\delta > 0$.
   (b) Two-sided test: H_1: $\delta \neq 0$.

Table 7.2 30 volunteer participants' weights data before and after 2 months with a diet pill (kg)

Number	Before	After	Number	Before	After
1	105	99.00	16	85	93.00
2	109	113.00	17	88	94.00
3	73	65.00	18	123	118.00
4	115	110.00	19	130	117.00
5	88	92.00	20	104	103.00
6	93	97.00	21	86	92.00
7	92	96.00	22	128	117.00
8	102	99.00	23	108	106.00
9	107	104.00	24	98	105.00
10	88	95.00	25	118	113.00
11	102	100.00	26	137	120.00
12	113	107.00	27	73	86.00
13	79	97.00	28	100	99.00
14	79	83.00	29	100	97.00
15	89	92.00	30	103	99.00

3. Choose α level (the confident level of the test is $(1 - \alpha)\%$).
4. The test statistic is

$$t = \frac{\bar{d}}{S_d / \sqrt{n}},$$ (7.3)

where

$$S_d = \sqrt{\frac{\sum d^2 - \frac{(\sum d)^2}{n}}{n-1}}$$ (7.4)

and the degrees of freedom is $\nu = n - 1$.

5. Make a decision based on the P-value (rejection rule). Reject the null hypothesis if:

(a) One-sided test: if $t \geq t_{\alpha,n-1}$ or if $t \leq -t_{\alpha,n-1}$.
(b) Two-sided test: if $|t| \geq t_{\alpha/2,n-1}$ (i.e., if $t \leq -t_{\alpha/2,n-1}$ or $t \geq t_{\alpha/2,n-1}$).

The sample size is $n = 30$, the difference mean is $\bar{d} = 0.2333$(kg) with a standard deviation $S_d = 7.5598$(kg).

The null hypothesis is essentially asking the question: "is the diet pill effective for losing weight?" and is tested as follows:

1. The null hypothesis H_0: $\mu_d = 0$.
2. The alternative hypothesis is one-sided test H_1: $\mu_d < 0$ (the diet pill is effective for losing weight).
3. The α level is 0.05.
4. The test statistic is

$$t = \frac{\bar{d}}{S_d / \sqrt{n}} = \frac{0.2333}{7.5598 / \sqrt{30}} = 0.1690.$$

5. Rejection rule: Reject H_0 if $|t| \leq |t_{0.05,29}|$; otherwise, H_0 could not be rejected. Since $t_{0.05,29} = 1.699$, $t < t_{0.05,29}$, the null hypothesis cannot be rejected. So, the pill is ineffective for losing weight.

7.5 Two-Sample t-Test

The two-sample (independent groups) t-test is used to determine whether the unknown means of two populations are different from each other, based on independent samples from each population. If the two sample means are sufficiently different from each other, then the population means are declared to be different. A related test, the paired t-test (discussed in the next section), is used to compare two population means using paired samples. The samples for a two-sample t-test can be obtained from two separate populations (e.g., male and female) or from a single population that has been randomly divided into two subgroups, with each subgroup subjected to one of two treatments (e.g., two medications). In either case, the two-sample t-test is only valid if the two samples are independent (i.e., unrelated to each other).

Suppose samples have been taken for the same variable from two independent groups, and it is necessary to determine whether the population means of the two groups are different.

To test whether the means for the two groups differ, a value for the t-statistic can be obtained using the following equations:

$$t = \frac{\overline{X}_1 - \overline{X}_2}{S_{\overline{X}_1 - \overline{X}_2}} \tag{7.5}$$

$$S_{\overline{X}_1 - \overline{X}_2} = \sqrt{S_c^2 \left(\frac{1}{n_1} + \frac{1}{n_2} \right)}, \tag{7.6}$$

where $\overline{X}_1$ and $\overline{X}_2$ are sample estimates of the population means (μ_1 and μ_2) for groups 1 and 2, respectively. $S_{\overline{X}_1 - \overline{X}_2}$ is the estimate of the standard error of the difference between the sample means ($\overline{X}_1 - \overline{X}_2$). S_1^2 and S_2^2 are the sample estimates of the variances (σ_1^2 and σ_2^2) of groups 1 and 2, respectively. n_1 and n_2 are the sample sizes for groups 1 and 2, respectively. S_c^2 is an estimate of the combined variance σ^2 if the variances of the two groups are assumed to be equal and can be obtained using the following equation:

$$S_c^2 = \frac{(n_1 - 1)S_1^2 + (n_2 - 1)S_2^2}{n_1 + n_2 - 2}. \tag{7.7}$$

When comparing two independent samples, the following assumptions must hold

1. The two samples must be independent from each other.
2. The individual measurements must be roughly normally distributed.
3. The variances in the two populations must be nearly equal.

Testing for the difference of the means of two independent samples (assuming equal variances) proceeds as follows:

1. State the null hypothesis and alternative hypothesis.

   (a) Two-sided tests: H_0: $\mu_1 = \mu_2$

   $$H_1 : \mu_1 \neq \mu_2.$$

   (b) One-sided tests: H_0: $\mu_1 = \mu_2$

   $$H_1 : \alpha_1 \langle \alpha_2 \text{ or } H_1 : \alpha_1 \rangle \alpha_2.$$

2. Choose α level (usually $\alpha = 0.05$).
3. Make a decision based on the *P*-value (rejection rule). Based on the observed value of *t*, reject the null hypothesis if:

(a) One-sided tests: if $t \geq t_{\alpha, n1 + n2-2}$ or if $t \leq - t_{\alpha, n1 + n2-2}$
(b) Two-sided tests: if $|t| \geq t_{\alpha/2, n1 + n2-2}$ (i.e., if $t \leq - t_{\alpha/2, n1 + n2-2}$ or $t \geq t_{\alpha/2, n1 + n2-2}$)

Example 7.3 To study the effect of new drug A on reducing blood glucose, a randomized controlled trial was conducted in a hospital with 66 patients who had type 2 diabetes mellitus. The patients were randomly divided into the trial group with sample size $n_1 = 30$ (using drug A) and control group with sample size $n_2 = 36$ (using Acarbose capsules); the fasting blood glucose was measured before and after 8 weeks, respectively; and the decrease of fasting blood glucose was shown in Table 7.3, differences of blood glucose is the fasting blood glucose decrease before and after 8 weeks for the two groups. Can we draw the conclusion that the fast blood glucose decrease effect of the new drug A and Acarbose capsules was different?

Consider the comparison of the fasting blood glucose decrease levels between new drug A and Acarbose capsules for type 2 diabetes mellitus, and the population mean of fasting blood glucose decrease effect for new drug A is assumed to be μ_1, while the mean of fasting blood glucose decreases for Acarbose capsules be μ_2. A comparison of these unknown means is performed by taking two samples of sizes $n_1 = 30$ and $n_2 = 36$ from the two populations.

Table 7.3 Fasting blood glucose decrease before and after 8 weeks for the trial group (drug A – group 1) and control group (Acarbose capsules – group 2) (mmol/L)

Group	Differences of blood glucose	Group	Differences of blood glucose	Group	Differences of blood glucose	Group	Differences of blood glucose
1	−0.70	1	3.25	2	2.17	2	2.00
1	1.65	1	3.50	2	1.65	2	2.05
1	2.00	1	4.28	2	2.00	2	2.00
1	2.91	1	2.50	2	2.91	2	1.28
1	0.90	1	2.75	2	1.90	2	1.30
1	3.50	1	3.50	2	3.50	2	4.50
1	5.80	1	2.90	2	3.70	2	1.70
1	0.80	1	3.70	2	1.35	2	−0.50
1	2.96	1	2.60	2	5.00	2	−0.79
1	2.71	1	2.50	2	2.20	2	1.01
1	3.65	1	4.80	2	0.80	2	2.29
1	2.75	1	2.40	2	0.20	2	1.12
1	5.95			2	0.60	2	3.88
1	4.83			2	2.10	2	4.20
1	2.34			2	0.60	2	0.66
1	2.85			2	−0.10	2	1.36
1	2.93			2	1.20	2	3.16
1	2.01			2	2.11	2	2.38

In this case, with two independent samples, consider the following issues:

1. The two sets of measurements are independent because the two sets with different treatments.

    (e.g., new drug A and Acarbose capsules).
2. In contrast to the one-sample case, two population means are simultaneously being estimated, instead of one. As a result, there are now two sources of variability, one from each sample.

In this example, $n_1 = 30$, $n_2 = 36$, $\overline{X}_1 = 2.9507$ (mmol/L), $S_1 = 1.3756$ (mmol/L), $\overline{X}_2 = 1.8747$ (mmol/L), and $S_2 = 1.35217$ (mmol/L).

Based on the two samples, the combined estimate of the population variance is

$$S_c^2 = \frac{(n_1-1)S_1^2 + (n_2-1)S_2^2}{n_1 + n_2 - 2} = \frac{(30-1)1.3756^2 + (36-1)1.35217^2}{30+36-2} = \frac{118.848}{64} = 1.857$$

The hypothesis test is carried out as follows:

1. State the null hypothesis H_0: $\mu_1 = \mu_2$.
2. Set up the two-sided alternative hypothesis H_1: $\mu_1 \neq \mu_2$.
3. The α level is 0.05 (the confident level of the test is 95%).
4. The test statistic is:

$$t = \frac{\overline{X}_1 - \overline{X}_2}{S_{\overline{X}_1 - \overline{X}_2}} = \frac{\overline{X}_1 - \overline{X}_2}{\sqrt{S_c^2\left(\frac{1}{n_1} + \frac{1}{n_2}\right)}} = \frac{2.9507 - 1.8747}{\sqrt{1.857^2\left(\frac{1}{30} + \frac{1}{36}\right)}} = 3.1938.$$

5. Make a decision based on the P-value (rejection rule). Reject H_0, if $t > = t_{\alpha/2,\ n1 + n2-2} = t_{0.05,64}$ or if $t < = -t_{0.05,64}$. Since $t_{0.05,64} = 2.00$, $t = 3.1938 > 2.000$, the null hypothesis is rejected.

In other words, we are 95% sure that type 2 diabetes mellitus with new drug A have significantly different fasting blood glucose decrease compared to Acarbose capsules.

7.6 The F Test for Equal Variances of Two Groups of Data

Another consideration that should be addressed before using the two-sample t-test is whether the population variances can be considered equal. An F-test is used to test whether the standard deviations of two populations are equal. This test can be either a two-tailed test or a one-tailed test. The two-tailed test against the alternative test states that the standard deviations are not equal. The one-tailed test only examines in one direction—the standard deviation of the first population is either greater than or less than the standard deviation of the second population. The choice is determined by the actual question. For example, if a new process is being tested, researchers may only be interested in knowing whether the new process is less variable than the old process.

F is the ratio of variances (the largest is the numerator) from samples of size n_1 and n_2. The degrees of freedom are $n_1 - 1$ and $n_2 - 1$, corresponding to sample variances of the numerator and denominator.

Only the upper tail probability needs to be considered, because the larger variance is always used as the numerator in the variance ratio F.

The F hypothesis test is defined as:

Null hypothesis H_0: $\sigma_1^2 = \sigma_2^2$;
Alternative hypothesis H_1: $\sigma_1^2 > \sigma_2^2$ for an upper one-tailed test.

Test Statistic $F = S_1^2 / S_2^2$, where S_1^2 and S_2^2 are the sample variances. The more this ratio deviates from 1, the stronger the evidence for unequal population variances.

Significance level $\alpha = 0.05$.

If only the F-value is available, then compare this value of F with the critical value ($F_{\alpha; \nu_1, \nu_2}$) of F for a selected level of significance, and ν_1 and ν_2 degrees of freedom [Appendix: F Distribution (homogeneity test of variances)].

If $F \geq F_{\alpha; \nu_1, \nu_2}$, reject H_0 and claim H_1.
If $F < F_{\alpha; \nu_1, \nu_2}$, do not reject H_0.

If the probability, Prob(F), for Levene's test is available, compare it with a selected significance level (α).

If Prob(F) $\leq \alpha$, reject H_0 and claim H_1.
If Prob(F) $> \alpha$, do not reject H_0.

A decision made on the basis of the foregoing criteria has the following consequences:

- **Equal Variances Assumed**. If H_0 cannot be rejected, assume that the variances, σ_1^2 and σ_2^2, are equal.

  - Use the *t*-statistic based on the pooled variances estimate to test whether the group means (μ_1 and μ_2) differ significantly.

- **Equal Variances Not Assumed**. If H_0 is rejected, and claim that H_1 is ($\sigma_1^2 \neq \sigma_2^2$), then one cannot assume the variances, σ_1^2 and σ_2^2, are equal.

  - Use the *t*-statistic based on separate variance estimates to test whether the group means, μ_1 and μ_2, differ significantly.

7.7 Two Types of Error and Power

7.7.1 Type I Error and Type II Error

In a hypothesis test, a type I error occurs when the null hypothesis is rejected when it is in fact true (i.e., H_0 is wrongly rejected). For example, in a clinical trial of a new drug, the null hypothesis might state that the new drug is no better than the current drug (H_0: There is no difference between the two drugs on average). A type I error would occur if it is concluded that the two drugs produced different effects when there was in fact no difference between them.

A type I error is often considered to be more serious and therefore more important to avoid than a type II error. Thus, the hypothesis test procedure is adjusted so that there is a guaranteed "low" probability of rejecting the null hypothesis wrongly (this probability is never 0). The probability of a type I error can be precisely computed as:

$$P(\text{type I error}) = \text{significance level} = \alpha$$

In a hypothesis test, a type II error occurs when the null hypothesis is not rejected when it is in fact false. For example, in a clinical trial of a new drug, the null hypothesis might state that the new drug is no better than the current drug (H_0: there is no difference between the two drugs on average).

A type II error would occur if it was concluded that the two drugs produced the same effect (i.e., there is no difference between the two drugs), when in fact they produced different ones. A type II error is frequently due to sample sizes being too small. The probability of a type II error is generally unknown but is symbolized by β and written as:

$$P(\text{type II error}) = \beta$$

Table 7.4 presents a summary of possible results for the hypothesis tests.

For any given set of data, type I and type II errors are inversely related. The smaller the risk of one error, the higher the risk of the other error.

Table 7.4 Summary of possible results for hypothesis tests

		Decision	
		Reject H_0	Accept H_0
Truth	H_0	Type I error	Right decision
	H_1	Right decision	Type II error

7.7.2 Power

The power of a statistical hypothesis test measures the test's ability to reject the null hypothesis when it is actually false—that is, to make a correct decision. In other words, the power of a hypothesis test is the probability of not committing a type II error. It is calculated by subtracting the probability of a type II error from 1, usually expressed as:

$$\text{Power} = 1 - P(\text{type II error}) = 1 - \beta \qquad (7.8)$$

The maximum power of a test is 1, and the minimum is 0. Ideally, a test should have a high power close to 1; usually, a power of 0.80 is acceptable for a statistical test.

7.8 Applications

There are three *t*-tests procedures in SPSS.

1. *One-sample t-tests* are used to check whether the mean of a single variable differs from a specified value.
2. *Two-sample t-tests* (independent-samples *t*-test) are employed to compare the means of particular variables between two groups.
3. *Paired-sample t-tests* are used to compare a pair of variables by checking whether the mean of the differences for the two variables is zero. It is appropriate for two types of studies: (1) measurements taken from the same individuals (e.g., measured before and after treatment); and (2) subjects matched in pairs at baseline with one member of each pair randomly assigned to the different groups.

7.8.1 One-Sample t-Test

Test the hypothesis that the mean pulse of a healthy adult man in mountainous area is equal to 72 times/min. First of all, transform the data above into an SPSS file. From the menu, choose (Fig. 7.1):

$$Analyze \rightarrow Compare\ Means \rightarrow One-Sample\ T\ test$$

7.8.1.1 Selected Output

See Fig. 7.2.

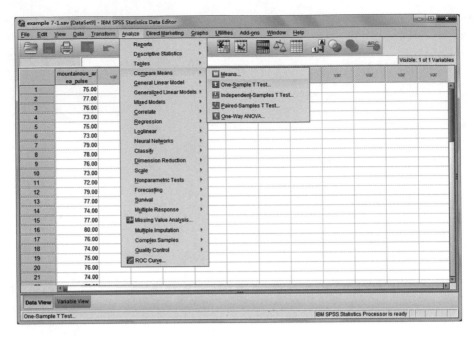

Fig. 7.1 Enter one-sample T test model

One-Sample Test

	Test Value = 72					
					95% Confidence Interval of the Difference	
	t	df	Sig. (2-tailed)	Mean Difference	Lower	Upper
mountainous_area_pluse	12.652	35	.000	3.91667	3.2882	4.5451

Fig. 7.2 SPSS output for one-sample test

7.8.1.2 Explanation

When a one-sample t-test is performed, the two-tailed significance (P-value) is smaller than $\alpha = 0.05$. Therefore, the null hypothesis is rejected, so the mean pulse of healthy adult males in a mountainous area population is different from the healthy adult male population with mean 72 times/min.

The 95% confidence interval of the difference is given in the last two columns. The 95% CI is (3.2882, 4.5451), which does not contain the point 0, so the null hypothesis at the 5% significance level should be rejected.

7.8.2 Paired-Sample t-Test

Test for the difference in weights (kg) before and after taking diet pills using a paired-samples t-test.

Paired Samples Test

| | Paired Differences | | | | | | | |
| | | | | 95% Confidence Interval of the Difference | | | | |
	Mean	Std. Deviation	Std. Error Mean	Lower	Upper	t	df	Sig. (2-tailed)
Pair 1 before - after	.23333	7.55980	1.38022	−2.58954	3.05621	.169	29	.867

Fig. 7.3 SPSS output for paired-sample *T* test

From the menu, choose:

$$Analyze \rightarrow Compare\ Means \rightarrow Paired - Samples\ T\ test.$$

7.8.2.1   Selected Output

See Fig. 7.3.

7.8.2.2   Explanation

The $P = 0.867$ is bigger than 0.05. It can be concluded that there is no difference in means for the weights before and after taking diet pills at the 5% level of significance.

7.8.3   Two-Sample **T**-Test

Conduct an independent samples *t*-test to compare the mean hypoglycemic effect of new drug A and Acarbose capsules for two independent groups of cases.
From the menu, choose:

$$Analyze \rightarrow Compare\ Means \rightarrow Independent - Samples\ T\ test$$

Select the dependent variable(s) that you want to test by clicking on it in the left hand pane of the independent samples *t* test dialog box. Then click on the upper arrow button to move the variable into the test variable(s) pane. In this example, move the hypoglycemia variable into the test variables box and the group variable into the grouping variables box. You need to tell SPSS how to define the two groups.

7.8.3.1   Selected Output

See Fig. 7.4.

Independent Samples Test

		Levene's Test for Equality of Variances		t-test for Equality of Means						
									95% Confidence Interval of the Difference	
		F	Sig.	t	df	Sig. (2-tailed)	Mean Difference	Std. Error Difference	Lower	Upper
hypoglycemia	Equal variances assumed	.095	.759	3.194	64	.002	1.07594	.33690	.40291	1.74898
	Equal variances not assumed			3.189	61.477	.002	1.07594	.33744	.40130	1.75059

Fig. 7.4 SPSS output for the independent samples test

7.8.3.2 Explanation

First, check the *P*-value of Levene's test for equality of variances. If this test is not significant, consult the first row (i.e., *Equal variances assumed*) of the *t*-test results; otherwise, consult the second row (i.e., *Equal variances not assumed*). Since the *P*-value of Levene's test is 0.759, which is bigger than 0.05, the variances of the two groups are equal. Therefore, consult results from the first row of the *t*-test. The *P*-value is 0.002, which is smaller than 0.05. It can then be concluded that there is difference between mean hypoglycemic effect of new drug A and Acarbose capsules at the 0.05 level of significance.

Chapter Summary
1. Hypothesis testing is a rational framework for applying statistical tests. Similar to estimation and confidence limits, the purpose of a hypothesis test is to permit generalization from a sample to the population from which it came. Both statistical hypothesis testing and estimation make certain assumptions about the population and then use probabilities to estimate the likelihood of the results obtained in the sample.
2. Steps in hypothesis testing: (1) Specify the null and alternative hypotheses and choose α. (2) Plot the frequencies of the two samples' basic data to check for normality. (3) In light of the assumption about variances, choose the appropriate test form. (4) Look up the critical value from the corresponding statistical table for the chosen α. (5) Calculate the statistic using the appropriate equation that will include the appropriate standard error calculation, and determine degrees of freedom. (6) Make a decision to either reject or fail to reject the null hypothesis.
3. The *t*-tests are used for testing difference between two means. The three types of *t*-tests discussed in this chapter are:

    (a) One-sample *t*-tests are used to compare a single mean to a fixed number or "gold standard."
    (b) Two-sample *t*-tests are employed to compare two population means based on independent samples from the two populations or groups.
    (c) Paired-samples *t*-tests are used to compare the difference mean between two samples from the paired groups in some way with zero.

Chapter 8
Analysis of Variance

Yupeng Wang, Qiuju Zhang, and Meina Liu

8.1 Introduction

This chapter introduces the first in a series of chapters devoted to linear models. The topic of this chapter, Analysis of Variance (ANOVA), provides a methodology for partitioning the total variance computed from a data set into components, each of which represents the amount of the total variance that can be attributed to a specific source of variation. The results of this partitioning can then be used to estimate and test hypotheses about population variances and means. In this chapter we focus our attention on hypothesis testing of means. Specifically, the testing of differences among means when there is interest in more than two populations or two or more variables is discussed. The techniques discussed in this chapter are widely used in the health sciences.

Experiments may be designed for single factor or multiple factors. The researcher can use different randomization procedures to accomplish the research work, such as completely random design, randomized block design, factorial design, split block design, repeated design, and so on. For different design strategy we can select different types of ANOVA. In this chapter we only introduce one-way ANOVA for completely design and two-way ANOVA for randomized block design.

Y. Wang · Q. Zhang · M. Liu (✉)
Public Health College, Harbin Medical University, Harbin, China

© Zhengzhou University Press 2024
X. Guo, F. Xue (eds.), *Textbook of Medical Statistics*,
https://doi.org/10.1007/978-981-99-7390-3_8

8.2   The Basic Idea of ANOVA

8.2.1   The Theme of ANOVA

Analysis of variance (ANOVA) is a commonly used statistical model for analyzing the relative contributions of identifiable sources of variation to the total variation in measured responses. In this method, the total variation of all the data can be divided into different parts (two or more) according to the study design, and it must include the random error. Then, compare the difference between the other parts of variation and the random error to determine whether there is statistical significance among the different group means.

Example 8.1 One experiment was conducted to estimate the association between exercise and bone health status, more exercise might make the bone become stronger. One researcher divided 30 rats into 3 groups randomly, 10 rats in each group. There were 3 treatments for different groups: no jumping for control group, low-jump treatment (the jump height was 30 cm, 10 jumps/day) for the experimental group one, high-jump treatment (the jump height was 60 cm, 10 jumps per day) for experimental group two. After 8 weeks the bone density (mg/cm³) of overall rats was measured. Please make the inference from the different means of three groups, whether the association between exercise and bone health exists or not.

This example is a completely random design, and we will use it to introduce the basic theory of ANOVA. According to 30 values in the Table 8.1, three kinds of variation can be obtained as follows:

1. Total Variation: The variation among 30 individual values, the variation between 30 values, and the overall mean, it represents the overall variation among the

Table 8.1 The bone density of the rats in the different groups (mg/cm³)

	Control	Low jump	High jump	Total
X_{ij}	611	635	650	
	621	605	622	
	614	638	626	
	593	594	626	
	593	599	631	
	653	632	622	
	600	631	643	
	554	588	674	
	603	607	643	
	569	596	650	
	10	10	10	
				30 ($SS_T = \sum\limits_{i=1}^{g}\sum\limits_{j=1}^{n_i}\left(X-\bar{X}\right)^2 = \sum\limits_{i=1}^{g}\sum\limits_{j=1}^{n_i}X_{ij}^2 - C$)
$\bar{X}_i$	601.1	612.5	638.7	617.4 ($\bar{X}$)

data, we called it Total Variation. It was denoted as MS_T (MS, mean square, shares the same meaning with variance S^2), it may be caused by treatment and random error.

$$SS_T = \sum_{i=1}^{g}\sum_{j=1}^{n_i}(X - \overline{X})^2 = \sum_{i=1}^{g}\sum_{j=1}^{n_i}X_{ij}^2 - C \tag{8.1}$$

$$MS_T = \frac{SS_T}{v_T} \tag{8.2}$$

$$v_T = N - 1 \tag{8.3}$$

where SS is the Sum of Squares, g is the number of groups, n_i is the number of individuals in each group, $\overline{X}$ is the overall mean, C is the correction index, v_T is the degree of freedom of total.

$$\overline{X} = \sum_{i=1}^{g}\sum_{j=1}^{n_i}\frac{X_{ij}}{N} \tag{8.4}$$

$$C = \left[\sum_{i=1}^{g}\sum_{j=1}^{n_i}X_{ij}\right]^2 / N \tag{8.5}$$

2. Variation of Between Groups: After 8 weeks for each group their group mean $\overline{X}_i$ is different, and they are also different with the overall mean $\overline{X}$, this variation we called it variation of between groups. It was denoted as MS_B, and it may be caused by treatment or random error.

$$SS_B = \sum_{i=1}^{g}n_i\left(\overline{X}_i - \overline{X}\right)^2 = \sum_{i=1}^{g}\frac{\left[\sum_{j=1}^{n_i}X_{ij}\right]^2}{n_i} - C \tag{8.6}$$

$$MS_B = \frac{SS_B}{n_B} \tag{8.7}$$

$$v_B = g - 1 \tag{8.8}$$

where v_B is degree of freedom of between groups.

3. Variation of Within Groups: The individual values in each group are different, and they are different with $\overline{X}_i$, this kind of variation we call it variation of within groups, it is caused by random error. It was denoted as MS_W or $MS_E = \frac{SS_E}{v_E}$.

$$SS_E = \sum_{i=1}^{g}\sum_{j=1}^{n_i}\left(X_{ij} - \overline{X}_i\right)^2 \tag{8.9}$$

$$MS_E = \frac{SS_E}{v_E} \tag{8.10}$$

$$v_E = N - g \tag{8.11}$$

where $\overline{X}_i$ denotes the mean of each group, v_E means the degree of freedom of within groups. And we can use the mathematical methods to prove that

$$SS_T = SS_B + SS_E \tag{8.12}$$

$$v_T = v_B + v_E \tag{8.13}$$

We can assume that if the exercise has no effect to bone health, three samples will share the same population, the difference among $\overline{X}_i$ is just caused by random error. In this condition the variation of between groups will be equal to the variation of within groups. Hence, both of them are caused by individual difference. Then the statistic F can be constructed.

$$F = \frac{MS_B}{MS_E} \tag{8.14}$$

This F value obeys F distribution with two degrees of freedom v_1 and v_2, which represents the difference between variation of between groups and variation of within groups, respectively. In theory, if the assumption of H_0 was true, then F value should be equal to 1; otherwise, it should be larger than 1. We can get conclusion according to the F value and F distribution.

8.2.2 Assumptions of ANOVA

Three important assumptions should be satisfied when applying ANOVA:

1. The observed values should be independent of each other;
2. The data in each group should follow normal distribution;
3. Homogeneity of variance, that is, the population variance of each group should be equal.

The assumption of normality concerns the sampling distribution of means; it is robust, especially when the sample size is large. Traditionally, Normality can be investigated by some statistical tools. The first one is calculating some indicators, such as Kurtosis coefficient and Skewness coefficient; the second one is the icon-method, such as Q-Q plot and P-P plot; third, the hypothesis test method also can be used to examine the distribution type.

For the assumption of homogeneous variances, Bartlett's test was commonly employed to make the conclusion.

8.2.3   Attentions

As we have seen, completely randomized design ANOVA may be used to test that g population means are identical; this is called one-way ANOVA. The null hypothesis should be:

$$H_0 : \mu_1 = \mu_2 = \mu_3 = \cdots = \mu_g$$

However, if we reject H_0, what happens? We can conclude that the population means are not all equal, but we cannot get the detailed information, we do not know whether all the means or only some of them are different. Once we reject the null hypothesis, we often want to conduct additional testing methods to find some detail information.

Under this condition, we may use the two-sample t-test mentioned in previous chapter. If we have three groups, we may conduct 3 times of t-test. However, we know that performing multiple tests will increase the probability of making type I error. We can avoid this problem by using some multiple comparison methods, such as LSD-t test, SNK-q test, Dunnett-t test, and so on.

If all the assumption conditions of ANOVA are satisfied, we can use the method directly. Otherwise, it will be necessary to do data transformation to meet the assumptions or select some other nonparametric testing methods.

8.3   One-Way Analysis of Variance

8.3.1   Completely Randomized Design

Completely randomized design is applied to estimate the effect of one primary factor with g ($g \geq 2$) levels. The level here refers to the possible status for the treatment factor. For example, drug can be a factor, and medicaments can be levels. Completely randomized design includes random grouping and random sampling.

Random grouping indicates N individuals are assigned into g treatment groups randomly, and sample size of each group can be same or different. If the sample size is equal in each group it is the balanced design; otherwise, it is unbalanced design. Random sampling means every individual in the population has the same probability to be selected. For completely randomized design, the levels of the primary factor are randomly assigned to the different group subjects, and then means were compared.

Example 8.2 One research team wanted to estimate the effect of a new drug for blood lipids, they conducted a double blind clinical research. 40 hyperlipemia patients were selected and assigned into 4 treatment groups randomly. Different groups received different treatment, group A received placebo, group B received a new drug with dose 2.4 g/day, group C received new drug with 4.8 g/day, group D received new drug 7.2 g/day. After 8 weeks the concentration of low-density lipo-

Table 8.2 Measures of LDL for subjects in four groups (mg/mL)

A: placebo	B: 2.4 g	C: 4.8 g	D: 7.2 g
3.53	2.42	2.86	0.89
3.30	1.98	2.32	1.74
1.37	2.36	2.41	2.16
2.33	2.27	2.28	3.37
3.53	2.93	3.64	1.27
4.34	2.34	2.66	1.41
3.59	3.11	3.04	1.92
4.00	2.22	2.81	1.69
3.52	3.57	1.97	1.19
2.96	1.81	2.65	2.11

protein (LDL) was measured for each patient. Please estimate the effect of the new drug (Table 8.2).

8.3.2 Variability Disassembly

According to the previous content were talked, for Completely Randomized Design the total variation can be divided into two parts, the Variation of Between Groups and Variation of Within Groups. $SS_T = SS_B + SS_E$, $v_T = v_B + v_E$. For this example, the variation between groups may be caused by the treatments, i.e. placebo, dose of 2.4 g, dose of 4.8 g, or dose of 7.2 g, or may be caused by individual difference. For the variation within groups is only due to the individuals difference.

The formulations of total variation, between groups variation, within groups variation and their corresponding degree of freedom, mean square, F value is settled in the following tables, that is one-way ANOVA Table 8.3.

8.3.3 Steps of ANOVA Analysis

Step 1: Data Structure (Table 8.4)

Step 2: Hypothesis
Null hypothesis, $H_0 : \mu_1 = \mu_2 = \ldots = \mu_g$

   Alternative hypothesis, H_1: not all the population means are equal.

   $\alpha = 0.05$, test is performed at the 0.05 level of significance.

   Null hypothesis implies all the population means are equal; in other words, any observed variation between the groups will be attributable to random sampling errors. Alternative hypothesis means at least one group mean is different from the others, or the difference is not attributable to random sampling errors if H_0 is rejected.

Table 8.3 One-way ANOVA table for completely randomized design

Source of variation	SS	DF	MS	F
Total variation	$SS_T = \sum_{i=1}^{g}\sum_{j=1}^{n_i}\left(X - \bar{X}\right)^2 = \sum_{i=1}^{g}\sum_{j=1}^{n_i}X_{ij}^2 - C$	$N-1$		
Between group	$SS_B = \sum_{i=1}^{g}n_i\left(\overline{X_I} - \bar{X}\right)^2 = \sum_{i=1}^{g}\dfrac{\left[\sum_{j=1}^{n_i}X_{ij}\right]^2}{n_i} - C$	$g-1$	$MS_B = SS_B/\nu_B$	MS_B/MS_E
Within group	$SS_E = \sum_{i=1}^{g}\sum_{j=1}^{n_i}\left(X_{ij} - \bar{X}_i\right)^2$ or $SS_T - SS_B$	$N-g$	$MS_E = SS_E/\nu_E$	

Table 8.4 The structure of data for completely randomized design

Number	Group 1	Group 2	...	Group g	
1	X_{11}	X_{21}	...	X_{g1}	
2	X_{12}	X_{22}	...	X_{g2}	
...	...	...	...	...	
n	X_{1n_1}	X_{2n_2}	...	X_{gn_g}	
n_i	n_1	n_2	...	n_g	N
$\bar{X}_i$	$\bar{X}_1$	$\bar{X}_2$	...	$\bar{X}_g$	$\bar{X}$

Table 8.5 The one-way ANOVA table

Source	Sum of squares, SS	Degrees of freedom	Mean square MS	F	Sig.
Groups (between groups)	SS_B	$\nu_B = g - 1$	$MS_B = SS_B/\nu_B$	MS_B/MS_E	P value
Error (within groups)	SS_E	$\nu_E = N - g$	$MS_E = SS_E/\nu_E$		
Total	SS_T	$\nu_T = N - 1$			

Step 3: Calculation of the Statistic

Usually, an ANOVA Table 8.5 will be used to illustrate the result of ANOVA.

ANOVA tests whether there are any differences between the groups with a single probability. Please note that several assumptions should be satisfied before an ANOVA is used.

Step 4: P-value and Conclusion

According to experiment and data analysis, make conclusion from two angles. The first one is statistical conclusion. According to the probability of null hypothesis to make the decision accept H_0 or reject H_0, then know whether the difference between groups is statistically significant or not. The second is clinical conclusion in terms of clinical knowledge.

8.3.4 Example

The information of Example 8.2 will be reused to introduce the whole procedure of one-way ANOVA.

A. Developing a hypothesis and setting significance level

Null hypothesis: $H_0 : \mu_1 = \mu_2 = \mu_3 = \mu_4$ the population means of four groups are equal.

Alternative hypothesis: H_1: not all the population means are equal.

$$\alpha = 0.05.$$

B. Calculating the relevant statistics (Table 8.6)

The overall mean is

$$\bar{X} = (3.25 + 2.50 + 2.66 + 1.78)/4 = 2.55$$

Total sum of observations and total sum of square observations are

$$\sum_{i=1}^{g}\sum_{j=1}^{n_i} X_{ij} = 32.47 + 25.01 + 26.64 + 17.75 = 101.87$$

Table 8.6 Measures of low-density lipoprotein for subjects in four groups (mg/mL)

	A: Placebo	B: 2.4 g	C: 4.8 g	D: 7.2 g
X_{ij}	3.53	2.42	2.86	0.89
	3.30	1.98	2.32	1.74
	1.37	2.36	2.41	2.16
	2.33	2.27	2.28	3.37
	3.53	2.93	3.64	1.27
	4.34	2.34	2.66	1.41
	3.59	3.11	3.04	1.92
	4.00	2.22	2.81	1.69
	3.52	3.57	1.97	1.19
	2.96	1.81	2.65	2.11
n_i	10	10	10	10
$\bar{X}_i$	3.25	2.50	2.66	1.78
$\sum X_i$	32.47	25.01	26.64	17.75
$\bullet\ X_i^2$	111.99	65.18	72.93	35.85

$$\sum_{i=1}^{g}\sum_{j=1}^{n_i}X_{ij}^2 = 111.99 + 65.18 + 72.93 + 35.85 = 285.95$$

$$C = \left(\sum_{i=1}^{g}\sum_{j=1}^{n_i}X_{ij}\right)^2 / N = (101.87)^2 / 40 = 259.44$$

N is total number of subjects, g is number of groups, n_i is number of cases within group i. The total sum of squares is

$$SS_T = \sum_{i=1}^{g}\sum_{j=1}^{n_i}X_{ij}^2 - C = 285.95 - 259.44 = 26.51$$

$$v_T = N - 1 = 40 - 1 = 39$$

k is number of groups. The sum of squares between groups is

$$SS_B = \sum_{i=1}^{g}n_i\left(\bar{X}_i - \bar{X}\right)^2 = \sum_{i=1}^{g}\frac{\left[\sum_{j=1}^{n_i}X_{ij}\right]^2}{n_i} - C$$
$$= \frac{32.47^2}{10} + \frac{25.01^2}{10} + \frac{26.64^2}{10} + \frac{17.75^2}{10} - 259.44$$
$$= 11.02$$

$$v_B = k - 1 = 4 - 1 = 3$$

$$SS_E = \sum_{i=1}^{g}\sum_{j=1}^{n_i}\left(X_{ij} - \bar{X}_i\right)^2 = SS_T - SS_B = 26.51 - 11.02 = 15.49$$

$$v_E = N - k = 40 - 4 = 36$$

The mean square between groups is

$$MS_B = \frac{SS_B}{v_B} = \frac{11.02}{3} = 3.67$$

The mean square error is

$$MS_E = \frac{SS_E}{v_E} = \frac{15.49}{36} = 0.43$$

Then the statistic index F ratio equals

$$F = \frac{MS_B}{MS_E} = \frac{3.67}{0.43} = 8.53$$

Table 8.7 The table of ANOVA

Source	SS	DF	MS	F	P-value
Treatment	11.02	3	3.67	8.53	<0.01
Error	15.49	36	0.43		
Total	26.51	39			

The results were settled into the ANOVA Table 8.7 as shown below.

C. Determining the P value

The P-value needs to be looked up in the F table [Appendix: F Distribution (analysis of variance)]; And a computer can give an actual value. In this example, if H_0 is true, the critical value of F ratio is 4.38 according to $\alpha = 0.01$ with $\nu_B = 3$ and $\nu_E = 36$ ($F_{0.01, 3, 36} = 4.38$). By comparing the actual $F = 8.53$ with the critical value $F = 4.38$, it can be concluded that the probability of null hypothesis being true is less than 0.01, null hypothesis should be rejected.

A significant F value indicates that there are differences in the means, but it does not tell us further information. If researchers want to know where the differences come from, or answer which treatment is most effective than others, it needs to do further analysis to judge the difference between the two groups using multiple comparisons.

8.4 Multiple Comparisons

It is easy to request a multiple comparison after the ANOVA test. In practice, when the difference among groups is significant, the researcher may be curious and want to know what the differences are. Is A better than B, C, and D? In general, after the null hypothesis of ANOVA has been rejected, the methods used to find the differences are called post-hoc tests, or multiple comparisons. They are pursued after the rejection of H_0 to identify the differences between any two groups. If H_0 was not been rejected, there is no need to take further post-hoc test.

There are a variety of multiple comparison tests to investigate the differences between two groups. For example, Duncan's multiple-range test, Student-Newman-Keuls test (SNK-q), least significant difference (LSD) test, Tukey's test, Scheffe's multiple-comparison procedure, and others. In this chapter, three commonly used methods of them will introduced, SNK-q test, LSD-t test, and Dunnett-t test. Other post-hoc tests can be found in references if necessary. The reason why we conduct special post-hoc test is to avoid the type I error and get the real conclusion.

8.4.1 SNK-q Test

If there are k groups, when researchers want to compare arbitrary two groups, $k*(k-1)/2$ times have to be taken, then one widely used method is the Student-Newman-Keuls test. In fact, it adjusts the final significant level at a specified value for each comparison by a q statistic.

Now back to Example 8.2. Supposed that before performing this experiment, researchers have already wanted to make some special comparisons. For example, researcher wonder if the new drug can decrease the value of low-density lipoprotein, then they can compare group A and B, A and C, A and D to see if there are really some differences between placebo group and drug groups. Researchers may also want to know if the low-density lipoprotein decreased with increase in dose, then they can compare group B with C, C with D, B with D to see if there are really some differences between different dose groups. Under this condition SNK-q test can be elected which is suitable for the comparison of arbitrary two groups.

The steps are as follows:

A. **Hypotheses** $H_0 : \mu_i = \mu_j$, $H_1 : \mu_i \neq \mu_j$, i and j denote groups, $\alpha = 0.05$.
B. **Test statistic**

$$q = \frac{\left(\bar{X}_i - \bar{X}_j\right)}{SE_{\bar{X}_i - \bar{X}_j}} \tag{8.15}$$

$$SE_{\bar{X}_i - \bar{X}_j} = \sqrt{\frac{MS_E}{2}\left(\frac{1}{n_i} + \frac{1}{n_j}\right)} \tag{8.16}$$

$$v = v_E$$

C. **P-value.** Use q table (Appendix: q Distribution) or statistical software.

For the data from Example 8.2, group A and D were compared as an example. The other comparisons will be done by SPSS in the application section.

A. **Hypotheses** $H_0 : \mu_A = \mu_D$, $H_1 : \mu_A \neq \mu_D$, $\alpha = 0.05$.
B. **Test statistic**

$$SE_{\bar{X}_D - \bar{X}_A} = \sqrt{\frac{MS_E}{2}\left(\frac{1}{n_i} + \frac{1}{n_j}\right)} = \sqrt{\frac{0.43}{2} \times \left(\frac{1}{10} + \frac{1}{10}\right)} = 0.3675$$

$$q = \frac{\left(\bar{X}_D - \bar{X}_A\right)}{SE_{\bar{X}_D - \bar{X}_A}} = \frac{1.7750 - 3.2470}{0.3675} = -4.01$$

$$v = v_E = 40 - 4 = 36$$

C. *P*-value.

$P < 0.01$, the probability from q table with DF of 36 indicates the population means between group A and D are statistically significant.

8.4.2 LSD-t Test

LSD stands for least significant difference test. It derives from the fact that you can determine the smallest difference as the critical value. If the actual difference is greater than that, then researchers can regard the result is statistically significant. It is different from the standard two-sample t-test, in this formula the mean square of error from ANOVA is taken to calculate the standard error of two sample means' difference. The LSD-t test is suitable for the comparison of one pair or several pairs which have some special professional meanings.

The steps are as follows:

A. **Hypotheses** H_0: $\mu_i = \mu_j$, H_1: $\mu_i \neq \mu_j$, i and j denote groups, $\alpha=0.05$.
B. **Test statistic**

$$t = \frac{\left(\bar{X}_i - \bar{X}_j\right)}{SE_{\bar{X}_i - \bar{X}_j}} \tag{8.17}$$

$$SE_{\bar{X}_i - \bar{X}_j} = \sqrt{MS_E\left(\frac{1}{n_i} + \frac{1}{n_j}\right)} \tag{8.18}$$

$$v = v_E$$

C. **P-value.** Use the normal t table or statistical software.

For the data from Example 8.2, group A and B are compared as an example. The other comparisons will be done by SPSS in the application section.

A. **Hypotheses.** $H_0 : \mu_A = \mu_B$, $H_1 : \mu_A \neq \mu_B$, $\alpha = 0.05$.
B. **Test statistic**

$$SE_{\bar{X}_B - \bar{X}_A} = \sqrt{MS_E\left(\frac{1}{n_i} + \frac{1}{n_j}\right)} = \sqrt{0.43 \cdot \left(\frac{1}{10} + \frac{1}{10}\right)} = 0.5198$$

$$t = \frac{\left(\bar{X}_B - \bar{X}_A\right)}{SE_{\bar{X}_B - \bar{X}_A}} = \frac{2.5010 - 3.2470}{0.5198} = -1.44$$

$$v = v_E = 40 - 4 = 36$$

C. *P*-value.

$0.10 < P < 0.20$, the 2-tailed probability from t table with DF of 36 indicates the population means between group A and B are not statistically significant.

8.4.3   Dunnett-t Test

The Dunnett-t test is computed exactly the same as LSD-t test, but a different t table of critical values is employed. It is suitable for the comparison of g-1 treatment groups with one control group. For example, you may only want to see if the drug is effective, then you can compare group A and B, A and C, A and D.

The steps are as follows:

A. **Hypotheses** H_0: $\mu_i = \mu_0$, H_1: $\mu_i \neq \mu_0$, i denotes experimental group and 0 denotes control group, $\alpha = 0.05$.
B. **Test statistic**

$$Dunnett - t = \frac{\left(\bar{X}_i - \bar{X}_0\right)}{SE_{\bar{X}_i - \bar{X}_0}} \tag{8.19}$$

$$SE_{\bar{X}_1 - \bar{X}_0} = \sqrt{MS_E \left(\frac{1}{n_i} + \frac{1}{n_0}\right)} \tag{8.20}$$

$$v = v_E$$

C. **P-value.** Use the special Dunnett-t table or statistical software.

For the data from Example 8.2, group A and B as an example will be compared, A is control group and B is one treatment group. The other comparisons will be done by SPSS in the application section.

A. **Hypotheses** H_0: $\mu_0 = \mu_B$, H_1: $\mu_0 \neq \mu_B$ $\alpha = 0.05$.
B. **Test statistic**

$$Dunnett - t = \frac{\left(\bar{X}_B - \bar{X}_0\right)}{SE_{\bar{X}_B - \bar{X}_0}} = \frac{2.5010 - 3.2470}{0.5198} = -1.44$$

$$SE_{\bar{X}_B - \bar{X}_0} = \sqrt{MS_E \left(\frac{1}{n_i} + \frac{1}{n_j}\right)} = \sqrt{0.43^* \left(\frac{1}{10} + \frac{1}{10}\right)} = 0.5198$$

$$v = v_E = 40 - 4 = 36$$

C. **P-value.**

$P > 0.05$, the probability from Dunnett-t table with 3, 36 of DF indicates the population means between A and B are not statistically significant.

8.5 Randomized Block Design ANOVA

Randomized block design ANOVA is a type of study design with one numerical outcome variable and two explanatory factors, one is treatment factor and the other is non-treatment factor (*block*), such as gender, weight, age, disease severity, and so on. Subjects are grouped by one such factor and the technical term for such a group is block.

For example, researchers may want to compare treatment effect by therapy and disease severity. If there are g levels for therapy and n levels for disease severity, different therapy is the treatment factor that we want to compare, and disease severity is the non-treatment factor (*block*) that may influence the treatment effect. Each block contains g observations which are randomly allocated, there will be a total of $N = g*n$ observations, simultaneously divided into n blocks with g observations in each and g groups with n observations in each.

Compared with completely random design, randomized block design divided the total variation into three parts: variation between treatments, variation between blocks, and variation of error. So it can disassemble some variation from primary "variation within groups" of completely random design and reduce the variation of error which will increase the statistical efficiency.

8.5.1 Randomized Block Design

Example 8.3 A study was conducted to compare the effect of three levels of digitalis work on calcium in the heart muscle of dogs. As we known the level of calcium uptake varies from different dogs, so it is better to select similar dogs in a block to keep a small difference within blocks. Then the researcher decided to select four different nests dogs, in each nest there are three dogs which will be randomly allocated into three levels of digitalis. The nest is regarded as block and the digitalis is regarded as treatment, the data of the three levels of digitalis (A, B, and C) are compared based on the heart muscle of 4 blocks in Table 8.8.

In this example, researchers want to explore if the level of digitalis affects the level of calcium in dogs. The analysis is similar with completely random design, but disassembling the variation into three parts.

Table 8.8 The effect of three levels of digitalis (nmol/L)

Nest	Levels of digitalis		
	A	B	C
1	1324	1608	1881
2	1140	1387	1698
3	1029	1296	1549
4	1150	1319	1579

8.5.2 Variability Disassembly

The variance (total sum of squares) is first disassembled into WITHIN and BETWEEN sums of squares. Between sum of square is then disassembled by intervention, blocking, and interaction. As randomized block design, there is no interaction between treatment and block.

The difference between completely random design and randomized block design is the variation of "block" factor. The particular formulas of randomized block design ANOVA are:

$$SS_T = SS_G + SS_B + SS_E \tag{8.21}$$

$$v_T = N - 1 \tag{8.22}$$

N is the total number of observations.

$$SS_B = \frac{1}{g} \sum_{j=1}^{n} \left(\sum_{i=1}^{g} X_{ij} \right)^2 - C \tag{8.23}$$

$$v_B = n - 1 \tag{8.24}$$

n is the number of blocks, g is the number of treatment groups.

$$SS_E = SS_T - SS_G - SS_B \tag{8.20}$$

$$v_E = (g - 1)(n - 1) \tag{8.21}$$

From the formula above, we can conclude that randomized block design can reduce variation of error and improve the ability to detect differences in treatments.

$$MS_G = \frac{SS_G}{DF_G} \quad MS_B = \frac{SS_B}{DF_B} \quad MS_B = \frac{SS_B}{DF_B} \tag{8.22}$$

The F value of treatments and F value of blocks are as follows:

$$F_G = \frac{MS_G}{MS_E} \quad F_B = \frac{MS_B}{MS_E} \tag{8.23}$$

If the variation between treatments (F_G) is large than 1.00, it means that the difference between treatments is not only caused by random error. Otherwise, meaning the difference is not statistically significant (Table 8.9).

8.5.3 Example

Example 8.4 One researcher selects randomized block design to compare the sarcoma inhibition effect of three kinds of drugs. First, 15 mice with sarcoma are matched into 5 blocks according to weight. Second, three mice in each block are randomly assigned into three treatment groups with different drugs. Change in weight is taken as the indicator to evaluate the effect of drugs. The question is whether the effects of three drugs are significantly different (Table 8.10).

A. Null hypothesis for treatments: $H_0 : \mu_1 = \mu_2 = \mu_3$
    Alternative hypothesis for treatments: H_1: The population of treatments is not all equal.
    Null hypothesis for blocking: $H_0 : \mu_1 = \mu_2 = \mu_3 = \mu_4 = \mu_5$
    Alternative hypothesis: H_1: The population of blocks is not all equal.

$$\alpha = 0.05$$

Table 8.9 The ANOVA table of randomized block design

Source	Sum of squares SS	Degrees of freedom DF	Mean squares MS	F	P-value
Group	SS_G	$\nu_G = g - 1$	$MS_G = SS_G/\nu_G$	MS_G/MS_E	P_G
Block	SS_B	$\nu_B = n - 1$	$MS_B = SS_B/\nu_B$	MS_B/MS_E	P_B
Error	SS_E	$\nu_E = (g - 1) \times (n - 1)$	$MS_E = SS_E/\nu_E$		
Total	SS_T	$\nu_T = N - 1$			

Table 8.10 The change in weight of mice after being treated with three kinds of drugs (g)

Block	Drug A	B	C	$\sum_{i=1}^{g} X_{ij}$	
1	0.82	0.65	0.51	1.98	
2	0.73	0.54	0.23	1.50	
3	0.43	0.34	0.28	1.05	
4	0.41	0.21	0.31	0.93	
5	0.68	0.43	0.24	1.35	
$\sum_{j=1}^{n} X_{ij}$	3.07	2.17	1.57	6.81	$\sum\sum X_{ij}$
$\bar{X}_i$	0.614	0.434	0.314	0.454	$\bar{X}$
$\sum_{j=1}^{n} X_{ij}^2$	2.0207	1.0587	0.5451	3.6245	$\bullet\bullet\ X_{ij}^2$

B. Test statistic

$$C = \left(\sum_{i=1}^{g} \sum_{j=1}^{n} X_{ij} \right)^2 / N = 6.81^2 / 15 = 3.0917$$

The total sum of square is

$$SS_T = \sum_{i=1}^{g} \sum_{j=1}^{n} X_{ij}^2 - C = 3.6245 - 3.0917 = 0.5328$$

$$v_T = N - 1 = 15 - 1 = 14$$

The sum of square of group is

$$SS_G = \sum_{i=1}^{g} \frac{\left[\sum_{j=1}^{n} X_{ij} \right]^2}{n} - C = \left(\frac{3.07^2}{5} + \frac{2.17^2}{5} + \frac{1.57^2}{5} \right) - 3.0917 = 0.2280$$

$$v_G = g - 1 = 3 - 1 = 2$$

The sum of square of block is

$$SS_B = \frac{1}{g} \sum_{j=1}^{n} \left(\sum_{i=1}^{g} X_{ij} \right)^2 - C$$

$$= \frac{1}{3} \left(1.98^2 + 1.50^2 + 1.05^2 + 0.93^2 + 1.35^2 \right) - 3.0917 = 0.2284$$

$$v_B = n - 1 = 5 - 1 = 4$$

The sum of square of error is

$$SS_E = SS_T - SS_G - SS_B = 0.5328 - 0.2280 - 0.2284 = 0.0764$$

$$v_E = (g-1)(n-1) = (3-1)(5-1) = 8$$

The mean square of group is

$$MS_G = \frac{SS_G}{v_G} = \frac{0.2280}{2} = 0.1140$$

The mean square of block is

$$MS_B = \frac{SS_B}{v_B} = \frac{0.2284}{4} = 0.0571$$

Table 8.11 The ANOVA table of randomized block design

Sources of variation	SS	DF	MS	F	P-value
Total	0.5328	14			
Group	0.2280	2	0.1140	11.88	<0.01
Block	0.2284	4	0.0571	5.95	<0.05
Error	0.0764	8	0.0096		

The mean square of error is

$$MS_E = \frac{SS_E}{v_E} = \frac{0.0764}{8} = 0.0096$$

Then the F value of group is

$$F_G = \frac{MS_G}{MS_E} = \frac{0.1140}{0.0096} = 11.88$$

Then the F value of block is

$$F_B = \frac{MS_B}{MS_E} = \frac{0.0571}{0.0096} = 5.95$$

The results are presented in the ANOVA Table 8.11 as shown below.

C. P-value.

By referring to F table, it can be found that $F_{0.05, 2, 8} = 4.46$, $F_{0.01, 2, 8} = 8.65$, $F_{0.05, 4, 8} = 3.84$, $F_{0.01, 4, 8} = 7.01$. For treatments $11.88 > 4.46$, so the null hypothesis should be rejected according to $\alpha = 0.05$, and H_1 is accepted. For blocks there is $5.95 > 3.84$, so H_0 of blocks should be rejected too, and H_1 is accepted. That means the effect of three drugs is significantly different, and the difference of mouse weights in blocks is statistically significant too. Note that researchers can use post-hoc test to compare different two groups.

8.6 Application

8.6.1 Example of One-way ANOVA

The data from Example 8.2 will be reused to illustrate how to perform one-way ANOVA by SPSS.

8.6.1.1   Build a SPSS Data File

There are two columns to present data. One column is the exact value of low-density lipoprotein and the other is group. The process of inputting the data into SPSS is File → Open → Data → select the data location or copy the text data file into SPSS. Then, we can determine the data type and the number of decimal places.

8.6.1.2   One-Way ANOVA by SPSS 20.0

The main process to show the one-way ANOVA by SPSS 20.0 is:
    Analyze → Compare Means → One-Way ANOVA → LDL → Dependent list → Group → Factor → Options → Post-Hoc → OK.
    Step by step process:

1. Analyze → Compare Means → One-Way ANOVA, enter One-Way ANOVA model, as shown in Fig. 8.1.
2. In One-Way ANOVA, we select the LDL value as Dependent, Group as Factor.
3. Click on Options: Select Descriptive, Homogeneity of variance test, Mean plot. Click on Continue.
4. Click on Post-Hoc: Select LSD method as multiple comparison method. Click on Continue, and then click on OK.

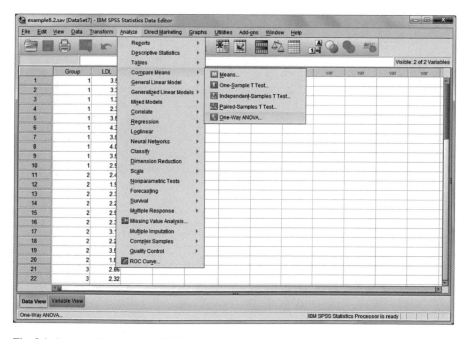

Fig. 8.1 Process of one-way ANOVA

8.6.1.3   Main Outputs of One-Way ANOVA by SPSS

Figure 8.2 descriptive table shows the information of mean, standard deviation, standard error, 95% confidence interval for mean, minimum, and maximum of each group.

Figure 8.3 shows the result of test of homogeneity of variances. The Levene's test for homogeneity of variance indicates that the P-value is greater than 0.05, so the variances of four treatment groups are not significantly different. It means the analysis of variance with the post-hoc comparisons can be used in a routine way. If the distributional assumptions of data were violated that means the data do not satisfy ANOVA, then it is need to resort to select the nonparametric method.

Figure 8.4 shows the ANOVA results. The F-test for "between groups" is 8.526, and *Sig* is <0.001 which is statistically significant. That means the four groups *are not all equal*, which indicates there are at least two groups are different. To identify which two groups are different, it is necessary to take post-hoc multiple comparisons.

Figure 8.5 shows the results of post-hoc multiple comparisons. In "group," 1, 2, 3, 4 indicate group A, B, C, D, respectively. According to the LSD test, except for A and C, B and C, all of the other groups have statistically different for means of low-density lipoprotein at the 0.05 level.

Descriptives

LDL

	N	Mean	Std. Deviation	Std. Error	95% Confidence Interval for Mean Lower Bound	95% Confidence Interval for Mean Upper Bound	Minimum	Maximum
1	10	3.2470	.85396	.27005	2.6361	3.8579	1.37	4.34
2	10	2.5010	.54071	.17099	2.1142	2.8878	1.81	3.57
3	10	2.6640	.46736	.14779	2.3297	2.9983	1.97	3.64
4	10	1.7750	.69503	.21979	1.2778	2.2722	.89	3.37
Total	40	2.5468	.82471	.13040	2.2830	2.8105	.89	4.34

Fig. 8.2 Descriptive table

Fig. 8.3 Outputs of homogeneity of variances test

Test of Homogeneity of Variances

LDL

Levene Statistic	df1	df2	Sig.
.780	3	36	.513

ANOVA

LDL

	Sum of Squares	df	Mean Square	F	Sig.
Between Groups	11.018	3	3.673	8.526	.000
Within Groups	15.508	36	.431		
Total	26.526	39			

Fig. 8.4 Outputs of One-ANOVA

Multiple Comparisons

Dependent Variable: LDL
LSD

(I) Group	(J) Group	Mean Difference (I-J)	Std. Error	Sig.	95% Confidence Interval	
					Lower Bound	Upper Bound
1	2	.74600*	.29352	.015	.1507	1.3413
	3	.58300	.29352	.055	-.0123	1.1783
	4	1.47200*	.29352	.000	.8767	2.0673
2	1	-.74600*	.29352	.015	-1.3413	-.1507
	3	-.16300	.29352	.582	-.7583	.4323
	4	.72600*	.29352	.018	.1307	1.3213
3	1	-.58300	.29352	.055	-1.1783	.0123
	2	.16300	.29352	.582	-.4323	.7583
	4	.88900*	.29352	.005	.2937	1.4843
4	1	-1.47200*	.29352	.000	-2.0673	-.8767
	2	-.72600*	.29352	.018	-1.3213	-.1307
	3	-.88900*	.29352	.005	-1.4843	-.2937

*. The mean difference is significant at the 0.05 level.

Fig. 8.5 Outputs of post-hoc multiple comparisons

8.6.1.4   Conclusion

The new drug with different doses has different effect in decreasing low-density lipoprotein value. The new drug with dose 2.4g and 7.2g per day has more effect in decreasing low-density lipoprotein value than placebo, but the new drug with dose of 4.8g per day is not significantly different compared to the placebo group.

8.6.2   Example of Completely Randomized Block Design ANOVA

We demonstrate the procedure of randomized block design ANOVA by using data of Example 8.4.

8.6.2.1 Build a SPSS Data File

There are three columns to present data of randomized block design ANOVA. The first column is the measurement of weight of 15 observations. The second is group, it means the drugs with a level of 1, 2, or 3 which indicates A, B, and C, respectively. The third is block with a level of 1, 2, 3, 4, and 5. The process of inputting the data into SPSS is File → Open → Data → select the data location or copy the text data file into SPSS. Then, we can determine the data type and the number of decimal places.

8.6.2.2 Randomized Block ANOVA by SPSS

The method to analyze randomized block ANOVA with the procedure by SPSS 20.0 should select general linear model (GLM), the main process is:

Analyze → General Linear Model → Univariate → Weight → Dependent Variable → Group, Bock → Fixed Factor(s) → Model → Options → Post-Hoc → OK.
Step by step process:

1. Analyze → General Linear Model → Univariate, enter Randomized block ANOVA model, as shown in Fig. 8.6.
2. In randomized block ANOVA model, we select the Weight value as Dependent, Group and Bock as Fixed Factors.

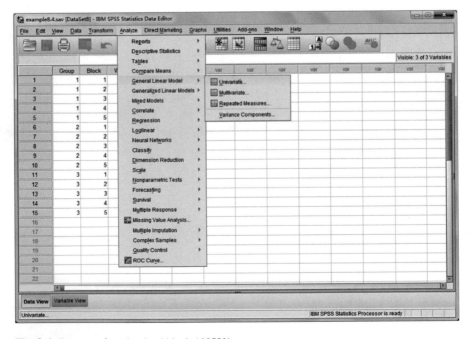

Fig. 8.6 Process of randomized block ANOVA

3. Click on Model: Click on Custom, Click on Build Term(s) and Select Main effects, Select Group and Block from "Factors & Covariates" part, and then move them to "Model" part. Click on Continue.
4. Click on Options: Select Group from "Factors and Factor interactions" part and then move it to "Display means for" part, Select Descriptive statistics. Click on Continue.
5. Click on Post-Hoc: Select Group from "Factors" part and then move it to "Post-Hoc Tests for" part, Select Bonferroni and S-N-K. Click on Continue, and then click on OK.

Bonferroni Correction

Bonferroni was developed by Carlo Emilio Bonferroni. It is a method of post-hoc test which changes the new significance level to avoid the type I error. It states that if a researcher tests n times of independent hypotheses on a set of data, then the new statistical significance level should be changed into α/n for each time separately, α is significance level, and n is the times of comparison. It is a safeguard against multiple tests of statistical significance on the same data.

8.6.2.3 Main Outputs of Randomized Block ANOVA

Figure 8.7 descriptive statistics provides some useful descriptive statistics including the mean and standard deviation for the dependent variable (weight) for each group*block, as well as all groups are combined (Total). These results can be used to describe data.

Figure 8.8 shows results of tests of between-subjects effects. This table gives us the main results of randomized block design ANOVA. In this table, it contains some information that is not necessary for the ANOVA, such as the rows headed Corrected Model (row 1), Intercept (row 2), and Total (row 6), those information can be ignored. The other rows are the standard ANOVA table for randomized block design. As expected, there is a significant difference between blocks (row 4, $F = 5.978$, $P = 0.016$) and also significant difference between groups (row 3, $F = 11.937$, $P = 0.004$). Because of the different decimal digits, this outcome is little bit different with Table 8.11.

Figure 8.9 shows the results of post-hoc multiple comparisons. In S-N-K table the value in subset is the means of three groups. Like "0.314" and "0.434" which are in the same column indicates these two groups have no difference statistically. Whereas "0.614" and "0.314" which are in different column indicates these two groups are statistically different.

Descriptive Statistics

Dependent Variable: Weight

Group	Block	Mean	Std. Deviation	N
1	1	.8200	.	1
	2	.7300	.	1
	3	.4300	.	1
	4	.4100	.	1
	5	.6800	.	1
	Total	.6140	.18420	5
2	1	.6500	.	1
	2	.5400	.	1
	3	.3400	.	1
	4	.2100	.	1
	5	.4300	.	1
	Total	.4340	.17097	5
3	1	.5100	.	1
	2	.2300	.	1
	3	.2800	.	1
	4	.3100	.	1
	5	.2400	.	1
	Total	.3140	.11415	5
Total	1	.6600	.15524	3
	2	.5000	.25239	3
	3	.3500	.07550	3
	4	.3100	.10000	3
	5	.4500	.22068	3
	Total	.4540	.19508	15

Fig. 8.7 Results of descriptive statistics

8.6.2.4 Conclusion

For the results of SNK-q test, the number presented is the mean of each group. If the means are presented in the same column, it indicates there are no significantly difference between groups, such as group B and C. Whereas if the means are presented in different column, they are significantly different, such as group A and B, A and C.

Tests of Between-Subjects Effects

Dependent Variable: Weight

Source	Type III Sum of Squares	df	Mean Square	F	Sig.
Corrected Model	.456[a]	6	.076	7.964	.005
Intercept	3.092	1	3.092	323.742	.000
Group	.228	2	.114	11.937	.004
Block	.228	4	.057	5.978	.016
Error	.076	8	.010		
Total	3.624	15			
Corrected Total	.533	14			

a. R Squared = .857 (Adjusted R Squared = .749)

Fig. 8.8 Results of between-subject effects tests

Multiple Comparisons

Dependent Variable: Weight

	(I) Group	(J) Group	Mean Difference (I-J)	Std. Error	Sig.	95% Confidence Interval	
						Lower Bound	Upper Bound
Bonferroni	1	2	.1800	.06181	.059	-.0064	.3664
		3	.3000*	.06181	.004	.1136	.4864
	2	1	-.1800	.06181	.059	-.3664	.0064
		3	.1200	.06181	.264	-.0664	.3064
	3	1	-.3000*	.06181	.004	-.4864	-.1136
		2	-.1200	.06181	.264	-.3064	.0664

Based on observed means.
The error term is Mean Square(Error) = .010.
*. The mean difference is significant at the .05 level.

Weight

	Group	N	Subset	
			1	2
Student-Newman-Keuls[a,b]	3	5	.3140	
	2	5	.4340	
	1	5		.6140
	Sig.		.088	1.000

Means for groups in homogeneous subsets are displayed.
Based on observed means.
The error term is Mean Square(Error) = .010.
a. Uses Harmonic Mean Sample Size = 5.000.
b. Alpha = .05.

Fig. 8.9 Results of multiple comparisons

8.7   Chapter Summary

1. Analysis of variance is one of the most commonly used statistical methods in comparing means among several groups. It aims to answer these two questions, which are: (a) is there a significant difference among several groups? (b) If so, which two groups are significantly different?
2. We should notice that check the distributional assumptions before using ANOVA is very important. If the distributional assumptions are violated, we should select to transform data so as to achieve normality or take some nonparametric tests as alternative.
3. The Basic Theory of ANOVA: The total variation of the all data can be divided into different parts (two parts or more than two parts) according to the study design, and it must include the random error. And then we compare difference between the other parts of variation and the random error to determine if there exists the significance or not among the different means.
4. After the null hypothesis of ANOVA has been rejected, it means that not all the groups are equal, but the result that every two groups are different cannot be concluded. So multiple comparisons should be taken to conclude which two groups are different. There are several post-hoc tests, each one has its' character, we should select appropriate methods under different situations.
5. Randomized block design ANOVA is the same as complete random design but with two categorical explanatory variables, one is treatment factor and the other is non-treatment factor (block). This kind of design divides total variation into three parts, it disassembles some variation from primary "variation within groups," so it can reduce the variation of error and will increase the statistical efficiency.

Chapter 9
Chi-Square Test

Yanxia Luo and Hongbo Liu

Objectives

Pearson's χ^2-test is one kind of hypothesis testing method for enumeration data using χ^2 values as a test statistic based on a χ^2 distribution. The χ^2 value reflects the deviation between the actual frequency (A) and theoretical frequency (T). The main purpose is to determine whether there are differences between a sample rate or proportion and the population rate or proportion. A χ^2-test can be conducted using SPSS software.

Key Concepts:

Chi-square test, Fourfold table, Contingency table, Theoretical frequency, Fisher's exact probabilities.

9.1 Introduction

When dealing with unordered categorical qualitative data, the counts are usually arranged in a tabular format known as a contingency table. A Chi-square test is a statistical procedure that compares frequencies or proportions in two or more groups using the information from a contingency table.

Y. Luo (✉)
School of Public Health, Capital Medical University, Beijing, China

H. Liu
School of Public Health, China Medical University, Shenyang, China

© Zhengzhou University Press 2024
X. Guo, F. Xue (eds.), *Textbook of Medical Statistics*,
https://doi.org/10.1007/978-981-99-7390-3_9

For example, a Chi-square test can be used to evaluate the effect of psychological counseling on disease prognosis in a sample of N individuals. In this example, there are two variables of psychological counseling and curative effect of disease prognosis and four combined frequencies (psychological counseling with effective curative effect; psychological counseling with inefficacious curative effect; non-psychological counseling with effective curative effect; non-psychological counseling with inefficacious curative effect). The information can be arranged into a contingency table and analyzed using a Chi-square test.

9.1.1 Chi-Square Distribution

The Chi-square distribution represents a type of continuous random variable probability function. If a random variable X_1, X_2, $\cdots$, X_n is mutually independent and obeys the standardized normal distribution, the distribution of the random variable $\chi^2 = \sum_{i=1}^{n} X_i^2$ should be the χ^2 distribution with the degrees of freedom of n. The graph of a Chi-square distribution is asymmetrical with only values greater than 0. Its shape relies on the degrees of freedom. With increasing degrees of freedom, the mean of the distribution moves more to the right (Fig. 9.1). The Chi-square distribution for df with α and its corresponding Chi-square value of $\chi^2_{\alpha, \nu}$ can be found in Chi-square critical value tables. Figure 9.2 shows us the Chi-square distribution critical value schematic diagram. The following rules can be concluded from the Chi-square critical value tables:

1. When the df is certain, there is an inverse relationship between the P-value and Chi-square critical value. As the P-value becomes smaller, the critical value becomes bigger.
2. When the P-value is certain, there is a direct relationship between the df and the Chi-square critical value. As the df becomes bigger, the critical value also becomes bigger.
3. When the df is 1, the P-value is certain, $\chi^2 = u^2$. The Chi-square critical value is equal to the square of u critical value.

Fig. 9.1 Chi-square distribution density probability plot ($df = 1,4,6,9$)

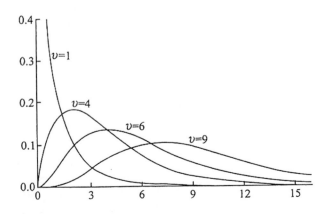

Fig. 9.2 Chi-square
distribution critical value
schematic diagram

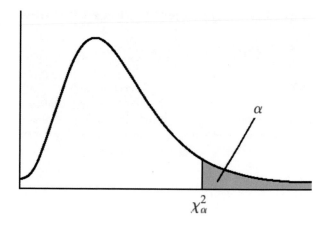

9.1.2 Basic Idea of Chi-Square Test

The Chi-square test was first proposed by statistician K. Pearson in 1899. The purpose is to test differences in rates or proportions. The main components are as follows:

H_0: There are no differences between the two population rates (or proportions).

H_1: There are some differences between the two population rates (or proportions).

The theoretical frequency is the expected value in a contingency table when H_0 is true. It can be calculated using the formula:

$$T_{ij} = \frac{n_i m_j}{n} \qquad (9.1)$$

where n represents the total number of cases, n_i represents the sum of the cases in row i, and m_j represents the sum of the cases in column j.

A Chi-square test statistic reflects the deviation between the actual frequency and theoretical frequency

$$\chi^2 = \sum_{i=1}^{R} \sum_{j=1}^{C} \frac{\left(A_{ij} - T_{ij}\right)^2}{T_{ij}} \qquad (9.2)$$

when H_0 is not true, there will obviously be a difference between the actual frequency and theoretical frequency. Therefore, the Pearson's χ^2 statistic will be bigger. When H_0 is true, the difference between the actual frequency and theoretical frequency will be smaller, so the Pearson's χ^2 statistic will be smaller.

The df can be calculated using the formula:

$$df = (R-1)(C-1) \qquad (9.3)$$

where R represents the number of rows and C represents the number of columns.

9.2 Two-Independent Samples Chi-Square Test

9.2.1 Data Format

Table 9.1 shows the basic 2 × 2 fourfold table.

There are four basic pieces of information (a, b, c, and d) in the table. The other data are all calculated from the four basic pieces of data; that is why this type of table in particular is called a fourfold table. These four pieces of information (a, b, c, and d) are known as the actual frequency.

9.2.2 Formulas

Formula 9.2 is useful for calculating the χ^2 value when the sample size, n, is greater than or equal to 40 and the theoretical frequency, T_{ij}, is greater than or equal to 5. Formula 9.2 is called the basic formula of a Chi-square test. A special formula can be derived from the basic formula to calculate the χ^2 value for a fourfold table.

The special formula for a Chi-square test of a fourfold table data:

$$\chi^2 = \frac{(ad - bc)^2 \cdot n}{(a+b)(c+d)(a+c)(b+d)} \tag{9.4}$$

when the sample size, n, is greater than or equal to 40, and the theoretical frequency is $1 \leq T_{ij} < 5$, Formulas 9.2 or 9.4 yield a bigger value for the statistic, which must be corrected. Britain statistician Yates F. reported corrected Chi-square values, which are referred to as a Chi-square with a continuity correction or a Chi-square with *Yates'* correction.

Continuity correction formula for a Chi-square test:

$$\chi^2 = \sum \frac{(|A - T| - 0.5)^2}{T} \tag{9.5}$$

Continuity correction formula for a Chi-square test of a fourfold table data:

$$\chi^2 = \frac{(|ad - bc| - 0.5n)^2 \, n}{(a+b)(c+d)(a+c)(b+d)} \tag{9.6}$$

Table 9.1 Chi-square 2 × 2 fourfold table

Treatment groups	Disease	No disease	Total
A	a	b	$n_1 = a + b$
B	c	d	$n_2 = c + d$
Total	$m_1 = a + c$	$m_2 = b + d$	$n = a + b + c + d$

when $n < 40$ (i.e., sample size) and theoretical frequency $T_{ij} < 1$, then an alternative procedure called Fisher's exact probabilities should be used for 2×2 tables. Although this method does not belong to the Chi-square test category, it can be supplementary to the Chi-square test.

The fourfold table of the four elements of a, b, c, and d is stochastic, since the total values of the rows and columns are fixed. The null hypothesis states that the observed frequencies or more extreme frequencies can occur by chance.

When H_0 is true with a fixed number of total values (row and column), the probability is:

$$P_i = \frac{(a+b)!(c+d)!(a+c)!(b+d)!}{a!b!c!d!n!} \tag{9.7}$$

where P_i represents the probability of the ith fourfold table, and a, b, c, and d are the four actual frequencies of the ith fourfold table.

The P-value of a statistical hypothesis test is "the probability of getting a value of the present or more extreme than that observed by chance alone, if the null hypothesis (H_0) is true.

9.2.3 Example

Example 9.1 A doctor wants to evaluate the effect of psychological counseling on the curative effect of disease prognosis. A total of 56 patients were randomly divided into two groups—one group received psychological counseling, while the other group was the control. All of the patients underwent the same pharmacological treatment. Try to appraise the curative effect of the psychological counseling treatment.

The results are given in Table 9.2.

Resolution
In Table 9.2, curative effect, including efficacy and inefficacy, is a qualitative variable. According to the data, efficacy was $20/28 = 71.43\%$ in the psychological counseling group and $15/28 = 53.57\%$ in the control group. The purpose was to test whether the population efficacy represented by the sample efficacy is equal. This problem can be solved by using a Chi-square test.

Table 9.2 Comparison of curative effects between two groups (Case number)

Groups	Efficacy	Inefficacy	Total
Psychological counseling	20	8	28
Control	15	13	28
Total	35	21	56

Hypothesis
$H_{0:}$ $\pi_1 = \pi_2$, the population efficacy represented by the two groups is the same.
 $H_{1:}$ $\pi_1 \neq \pi_2$, the population efficacy represented by the two groups is not the same.

$$\alpha = 0.05$$

Calculate the Statistic
The total sample size is 56, which is over 40, and the smallest theoretical frequency
is $T_{min} = \dfrac{28 \times 21}{56} = 10.5 > 5$. Therefore, use the special formula for a Chi-square test
for fourfold table data (Formula 9.4) to compute the statistic.

$$\chi^2 = \frac{(20 \times 13 - 8 \times 15)^2 \cdot 56}{28 \times 28 \times 35 \times 21} = 1.905 \quad df = 1$$

Calculate the P-value and Make a Conclusion
Looking at the Chi-square critical value table (Appendix: χ^2 Distribution),
$\chi^2_{0.05,\,1} = 3.84$, $1.905 < \chi^2_{0.05,\,1}$, so $P > 0.05$.

At the level of $\alpha = 0.05$, null hypothesis (H_0) cannot be rejected, since there is no
statistical significance between the two groups. This result suggests that there is no
significant difference of the efficacy between the treatment and control groups.

Example 9.2 It is thought that influenza vaccine can give greater protection against
infection in subjects with vaccinal vaccinate, since their immune system may
already have been "primed" by that earlier infection. In a study of the relationship
between influenza infection and the efficacy of an influenza vaccine, 78 subjects
were recruited and 52 vaccinated, and then followed through the following influenza season to determine new infections. The results are given in Table 9.3. Are
there different infected rates between subjects with and without vaccinal vaccinate?

Resolution
In Table 9.3, the result of infection, including infected and not infected, is a qualitative variable. According to the data, infected rate was 5/52 = 9.61% in the subjects
with vaccinal vaccinate and 8/26 = 30.77% in the subjects without vaccinal vaccinate. The purpose was to test whether the population infected rates represented by
the sample infected rates is equal. This problem can be solved by using a Chi-
square test.

Hypothesis
$H_{0:}$ $\pi_1 = \pi_2$, the population infected rates represented by the subjects with and without vaccinal vaccinate is the same.
 $H_{1:}$ $\pi_1 \neq \pi_2$, the population infected rates represented by the subjects with and
without vaccinal vaccinate is not the same.

$$\alpha = 0.05$$

Table 9.3 Comparison of infected rates between two groups (case number)

Status during follow-up	Infected	Not infected	Total
With vaccinal vaccinate	5	47	52
Without vaccinal vaccinate	8	18	26
Total	13	65	78

Calculate the Statistic

The total sample size is 78, which is over 40, and the smallest theoretical frequency is $T_{min} = \dfrac{26 \times 13}{78} = 4.33 < 5$. Therefore, use the continuity correction formula for a Chi-square test for fourfold table data (Formula 9.6) to compute the statistic.

$$\chi^2 = \frac{\left(|5 \times 18 - 8 \times 47| - 0.5 \times 78\right)^2 \cdot 78}{52 \times 26 \times 13 \times 65} = 4.165 \quad df = 1$$

Calculate the P-value and Make a Conclusion
Looking at the Chi-square critical value table (Appendix: χ^2 Distribution), $\chi^2_{0.05,\,1} = 3.84$, $4.165 > \chi^2_{0.05,\,1}$, so $P < 0.05$.

At the level of $\alpha = 0.05$, null hypothesis (H_0) cannot be accepted, since there is statistical significance between the two groups. This result suggests that there is significant difference of the infected rates in the subjects with and without vaccinal vaccinate.

9.2.4 Application of Software

1. The three variables from Example 9.1 were defined and input into SPSS.
2. Set up the frequency variable: Data → Weight Cases → Weight cases by → Move the frequency variable from the left frame to the right frame by clicking the right arrow button after selecting the appropriate variable. Click OK.
3. Analyze the data: Analyze → Descriptive Statistics → Crosstabs → Move the variables to be tested (group and effect) from the left frame to the right frame (Row(s)and Column(s)) by clicking the right arrow button after selecting the appropriate variables (as shown in Fig. 9.3).
4. Click on the Statistics button to open the window. Select "Chi-square." Click on the Continue button to return to the Crosstabs window. Click the OK button to run the test.
5. Main output results.

    Figure 9.4 displays the results analyzed by SPSS.

    How to select an exact result is very important. Firstly, we should identify two variables.

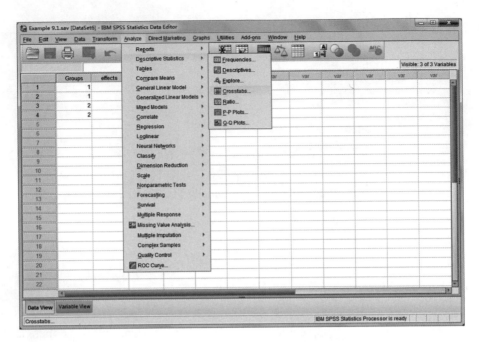

Fig. 9.3 Chi-square test with SPSS

Chi-Square Tests					
	Value	df	Asymp. Sig. (2-sided)	Exact Sig. (2-sided)	Exact Sig. (1-sided)
Pearson Chi-Square	1.905ᵃ	1	.168		
Continuity Correctionᵇ	1.219	1	.270		
Likelihood Ratio	1.919	1	.166		
Fisher's Exact Test				.269	.135
Linear-by-Linear Association	1.871	1	.171		
N of Valid Cases	56				
a. 0 cells (.0%) have expected count less than 5. The minimum expected count is 10.50.					
b. Computed only for a 2x2 table					

Fig. 9.4 Test statistics

The first variable is sample size, which is shown in the last line as "N of Valid Cases," in this case it is 56. The second variable is theoretical frequency (T), which is shown in the footnote as "b. 0 cells (.0%) have an expected count of less than 5. The minimum expected count is 10.50." With a sample size $n \geq 40$ and theoretical frequency $T_{ij} \geq 5$, the *Pearson* Chi-Square in Line 1 should be used (Example 9.1). With a sample size $n \geq 40$, but theoretical frequency $1 \leq T_{ij} < 5$, the continuity correction in Line 2 should be used (Example 9.2). With a sample size $n < 40$ or theoretical frequency $T_{ij} < 1$, the Fisher's exact test in Line 4 should be used. In this example, $n = 56 > 40$ and theoretical frequency $T_{ij} \geq 5$, so a Pearson Chi-square test should be used. In this case, $\chi^2 = 1.905$, $P = 0.168$, and $P > 0.05$.

6. Conclusion

$P > 0.05$, so at the level of $\alpha = 0.05$, H_0 cannot be rejected. The results suggested that there is no significant difference of the efficacy between the psychological counseling treatment group and control group.

9.3 Paired Design Chi-Square Test

9.3.1 Data Format

When the data are paired, rather than independent, McNemar's test can be used for comparing paired proportions. A fourfold table would be called a paired fourfold table. Table 9.4 shows the basic paired 2 × 2 fourfold table.

9.3.2 Formulas

McNemar's Test is generally used when the data consist of paired observations. When $b + c \geq 40$, Formula 9.2 can also be used to calculate the statistic. Since a, b, c, and d are all paired numbers, Formula 9.2 can be changed into Formula 9.8.

$$\chi^2 = \frac{(b-c)^2}{b+c} \qquad v = 1 \tag{9.8}$$

when $b + c < 40$, use Formula 9.4 to calculate the statistic by formatting Formula 9.2 into Formula 9.9.

$$\chi^2 = \frac{(|b-c|-1)^2}{b+c} \qquad v = 1 \tag{9.9}$$

Table 9.4 Paired design 2 × 2 fourfold table

Method A	Method B		
	+	−	Total
+	a	b	$n_1 = a + b$
−	c	D	$n_2 = c + d$
Total	$m_1 = a + c$	$m_2 = b + d$	$n = a + b + c + d$

Table 9.5 Results of testing sputum specimens using two different methods

Method A	Method B		Total
	+	−	
+	68	12	80
−	7	13	20
Total	75	25	100

9.3.3 Example

Example 9.3 A study evaluated whether there was a difference between using two kinds of methods to test the sputum specimen in 120 patients. The results are presented below (Table 9.5).

Resolution
In this study, each subject has been tested twice by two kinds of methods (A and B); the outcome is a binary (positive/negative) variable; and researchers want to know whether the positive rates are different between the methods A and B. The data are paired observations and McNemar's test can be used to analyze this type of study.

Hypothesis
H_0: $\pi_1 = \pi_2$, the positive rates tested by two kinds of methods are the same.
   H_1: $\pi_1 \neq \pi_2$, the positive rates tested by two kinds of methods are different.

$$\alpha = 0.05$$

Calculate the Statistic
In this example, $b + c = 12 + 7 = 19 < 40$, so Formula 9.9 can be used to calculate the statistic.

$$\chi^2 = \frac{(||12 - 7|| \ 1)^2}{12 + 7} = 0.842 \quad df = 1$$

Calculate the P-value and Make a Conclusion
Looking at the Chi-square critical value table, $\chi^2_{0.05, 1} = 3.84$ and $0.842 < \chi^2_{0.05, 1}$, so $P > 0.05$.

   At the level of $\alpha = 0.05$, H_0 cannot be rejected, since there is no statistical significance between the two groups. The results suggest that there is no significant difference of the positive rates tested by two different methods.

9.3.4 Application of Software

1. The three variables from Example 9.3 were defined and inputted into SPSS referring to Fig. 9.3.
2. Set up the frequency variable: Data → Weight Cases → Weight cases by → Move the frequency variable from the left frame to the right frame by clicking the right arrow button after selecting the appropriate variable. Click OK.

3. Analyze the data: Analyze → Descriptive Statistics → Crosstabs → Move the variables to be tested (*A* and *B*) from the left frame to the right frame (Row(s) and Column(s)) by clicking the right arrow button after selecting the appropriate variables.
4. Click on the "Statistics" button and Select "McNemar."
   Click "Continue" to return to the Crosstabs window. Click OK to run the test.
5. Main output results
   From Fig. 9.5, the *P*-value is obtained ($P = 0.359$).
6. Conclusion
   $P > 0.05$, so H_0 cannot be rejected. The results suggest that there is no signifi-cant difference of the positive rates tested by the two different methods.

9.4 Chi-Square Test for R × C Table

9.4.1 Data Format

When comparing the proportions of *R* groups of independent samples, the data can be arranged as an $R \times C$ contingency table, where *R* is the number of rows and *C* is the number of columns. There is at least one count of *R* or *C* over 2 (Table 9.6).

Fig. 9.5 Test statistics

Chi-Square Tests		
	Value	Exact Sig. (2-sided)
McNemar Test		.359[a]
N of Valid Cases	100	
a. Binomial distribution used.		

Table 9.6 $R \times C$ contingency table

Treatment groups	Attribute (or levels)				Total
	1	2	...	C	
Group 1	A_{11}	A_{12}	...	A_{1C}	n_1
Group 2	A_{21}	A_{22}	...	A_{2C}	n_2
...	...	...	...	...	...
Group R	A_{R1}	A_{R2}	...	A_{RC}	n_R
Total	m_1	m_2	...	m_C	n

9.4.2 Formulas

In a Chi-square test for $R \times C$ contingency tables, the theoretical frequency (T) cannot be smaller than 1. Moreover, any theoretical frequencies below 5 cannot exceed 1/5 of cells. Otherwise, the contiguous rows or columns must be combined with smaller frequencies to avoid throwing off the rows or columns with the smaller frequencies. Another alternative is to use Fisher's exact test. However, the best method is to increase the sample size.

Formula 9.2 can still be used when carrying out a hypothesis test, and the df can be calculated using Formula 9.3. A formula for $R \times C$ contingency tables can be derived from Formula 9.2 as the following formula (9.10).

$$\chi^2 = n \left(\sum_{i=1}^{R} \sum_{j=1}^{C} \frac{A_{ij}^2}{n_i m_j} - 1 \right)$$ (9.10)

where n is the total number, n_i is the total number in row i, m_j is the total number in column j, and A_{ij} is the actual frequency of row i and column j.

9.4.3 Example

Example 9.4 A clinical research group has conducted a study to relate the incidence rates of side effects associated with a new therapeutic agent and patient groups. The results of the study are as follows. Using an appropriate method to examine whether the incidence rates of side effects are equal in patient groups.

Resolution
In Table 9.7, there are four levels for patient groups (A, B, C, and D). The data were arranged in a 2×4 contingency table, and a Chi-square test for R × C contingency tables was conducted.

Hypotheses
H_0: The incidence rates of the side effects are the same in different patients.
    H_1: The incidence rates of the side effects are different in different patients.

$$\alpha = 0.05$$

Calculate the Statistic
The minimal theoretical frequency is $T_{min} = \dfrac{35 \times 64}{165} = 13.6 > 5$, so a Chi-square test for $R \times C$ contingency tables can be used to calculate the statistic.

Table 9.7 The side effects in different patients (case number)

Patient group (years)	With side effects	Without side effects	Total
A	8	28	36
B	16	23	39
C	15	20	35
D	25	30	55
Total	64	101	165

$$\chi^2 = 165 \times \left(\frac{8^2}{36 \times 64} + \frac{28^2}{36 \times 101} + \frac{16^2}{39 \times 64} + \frac{23^2}{39 \times 101} + \frac{15^2}{35 \times 64} + \frac{20^2}{35 \times 101} + \frac{25^2}{55 \times 64} + \frac{30^2}{55 \times 101} - 1 \right) = 5.517$$

$$df = (2-1)(4-1) = 3$$

Calculate the *P*-value and Make a Conclusion

Looking at a Chi-square critical value table, $\chi^2_{0.05,\,3} = 7.815$ and $5.517 < \chi^2_{0.05,\,3}$, so $P > 0.05$. At the $\alpha = 0.05$ level of significance, the null hypothesis (H_0) cannot be rejected and there isn't a statistically significant difference. The results suggest that the incidence rates of the side effect is the same in different patients.

Example 9.5 A study investigates whether the source of first aid knowledge is different in community populations with different occupations. The data are displayed in the form of a 3 × 4 contingency table (Table 9.8).

Resolution

In Table 9.8, there are three levels for the occupation variable (Cadre, Worker, and Others) and four levels for the source of first aid knowledge variable (Internet, TV or publication, Friends, and Others). The data were arranged in a 3 × 4 contingency table, and a Chi-square test for R × C contingency tables was conducted.

Hypotheses

H_0: The proportions of the sources of first aid knowledge are the same in different occupational populations.

H_1: The proportions of the sources of first aid knowledge are different in different occupational populations.

$$\alpha = 0.05$$

Calculate the Statistic

The minimal theoretical frequency is $T_{min} = \dfrac{277 \times 162}{978} = 45.9 > 5$, so a Chi-square test for $R \times C$ contingency tables can be used to calculate the statistic.

Table 9.8 Main source of first aid knowledge in different occupational populations (case number)

Occupation	Main source of first aid knowledge				Total
	Internet	TV or publication	Friends	Others	
Cadre	84	116	41	36	277
Worker	81	152	68	52	353
Others	42	136	96	74	348
Total	207	404	205	162	978

$$\chi^2 = 978 \times (\frac{84^2}{277 \times 207} + \frac{116^2}{277 \times 404} + \frac{41^2}{277 \times 205} + \frac{36^2}{277 \times 162} + \frac{81^2}{353 \times 207} + \frac{152^2}{353 \times 404}$$

$$+ \frac{68^2}{353 \times 205} + \frac{52^2}{353 \times 162} + \frac{42^2}{348 \times 207} + \frac{136^2}{348 \times 404} + \frac{96^2}{348 \times 205} + \frac{74^2}{348 \times 162} \quad 1)$$

$$= 46.088$$

$$df = (3-1)(4-1) = 6$$

Calculate the *P*-value and Make a Conclusion

Looking at a Chi-square critical value table, $\chi^2_{0.05, 6} = 12.59$ and $46.088 > \chi^2_{0.05, 6}$, so $P < 0.05$. At the $\alpha = 0.05$ level of significance, the null hypothesis (H_0) is rejected and there is a statistically significant difference. The results suggest that the proportions of the sources of first aid knowledge are significantly different in different occupational populations.

9.4.4 Application of Software

1. The three variables from Example 9.5 were defined and inputted into SPSS referring to Fig. 9.3.
2. Select the Weight Cases: Data → Weight Cases → Weight Cases By → Move the frequency variable from the left frame to the right frame by clicking the right arrow button after selecting the appropriate variable. Click OK.
3. Analyze the data: Analyze → Descriptive Statistics → Crosstabs → Move the variables to be tested (occupation and source) from the left frame to the right frame (Row(s) and Column(s)) by clicking the right arrow button after selecting the appropriate variables.
4. Click on "Statistics" to open the window and select "Chi-square." Click "Continue" to return to the Crosstabs window. Click OK to run the test.
5. Main output results

   In Fig. 9.6, the contingency table for the test is obtained.

   Figure 9.7 displays the results analyzed by SPSS.

occupation * source Crosstabulation						
Count						
		source				Total
		internet	TV or publication	friends	others	
occupation	cadre	84	116	41	36	277
	worker	81	152	68	52	353
	others	42	136	96	74	348
Total		207	404	205	162	978

Fig. 9.6 Descriptive statistics

Chi-Square Tests			
	Value	df	Asymp. Sig. (2-sided)
Pearson Chi-Square	46.088[a]	6	.000
Likelihood Ratio	47.030	6	.000
Linear-by-Linear Association	36.989	1	.000
N of Valid Cases	978		

a. 0 cells (.0%) have expected count less than 5. The minimum expected count is 45.88.

Fig. 9.7 Test statistics

With theoretical frequencies of $T_{ij} \geq 1$, and the number of theoretical frequencies of $1 \leq T_{ij} < 5$ that do not exceed 1/5 of the cells, the *Pearson* Chi-square formula shown in line 1 can be used.

When $T_{ij} < 1$, or the number of theoretical frequencies of $1 \leq T_{ij} < 5$ exceeds 1/5 of the cells, Fisher's Exact Test should be used. Click "Exact" in the "Crosstabs window" $\rightarrow$ Exact Tests window, Monte Carlo or Exact. Click "Continue" to return to the Crosstabs window. Click OK to run the test.

In this example, all of the theoretical frequencies $T_{ij} \geq 5$, so $\chi^2 = 46.088$, and $P < 0.001 < 0.05$.

6. Conclusion

Since $P < 0.05$ at the level of $\alpha = 0.05$, reject H_0. The results suggest that the proportions of the sources of first aid knowledge are significantly different in different occupational populations.

Chapter Summary

1. When working with qualitative data that have been grouped into categories, arrange the data in a contingency table, such as a 2×2 fourfold table, paired fourfold table, or $R \times C$ contingency table.
2. It is important to first check the total number and theoretical frequencies in order to choose an appropriate formula to conduct a Chi-square test.
3. When the null hypothesis is rejected in a Chi-square test for many independent sample frequencies and frequency distribution, it only means that the proportions are not all the same. In order to understand which ones are different, multiple comparisons must be carried out.
4. A Chi-square test for contingency table is not all purpose. For example, it is best to choose the method of a rank sum test for ordinal data, and a log-linear model and logistic regression model for multidimensional contingency table data.

Chapter 10
Nonparametric Tests

Hong He and Linlin Li

Objectives

Nonparametric tests involve testing whether the sampled data are from the same population when the population is not normally distributed or the underlying distribution is not known. Whether the population follows any kind of distribution is irrelevant, since the test does not depend on the underlying distribution. In fact, this testing method is not based on the comparison of parameters, but on the distributions. Therefore, nonparametric statistics make fewer assumptions about the nature of the underlying distributions. Furthermore, the statistical procedure of this method is both easy and convenient. As a result, nonparametric statistics are widely used, especially when there is not enough information.

Key Concepts:
Nonparametric statistics, rank, rank sum test

10.1 Introduction to Nonparametric Statistics

A nonparametric test is one of the most significant methods of statistical analysis, forming the basic content of statistical inferences together with parametric tests. Parametric methods are used to test the values of certain parameters (e.g., mean and

H. He (✉)
Institute of Health Science Research, School of Sociology and Population Studies, Renmin University of China, Beijing, China

L. Li
School of Public Health, Zhengzhou University, Zhengzhou, China

© Zhengzhou University Press 2024   141
X. Guo, F. Xue (eds.), *Textbook of Medical Statistics*,
https://doi.org/10.1007/978-981-99-7390-3_10

standard deviation) on the condition that the forms of the underlying distributions are known. In some cases, the definite form of the underlying distribution cannot be assumed; in other words, the data do not conform to the assumptions that the populations are normally distributed or approximately so. In this situation, parametric methods cannot be used. Instead, nonparametric methods, which make fewer assumptions about the nature of the underlying distribution, can be applied to test the distribution by using the sample data.

There are several advantages for using nonparametric test. First, nonparametric tests do not make assumptions about the underlying distribution of differences. In other words, the normally distributed data are not required, in which it is necessary for parametric tests. Second, nonparametric methods are also relatively simple, so they are easily understood and used. When the sample size is not large enough, especially when conducting a test without using computer software, nonparametric tests save time and labor. Nonparametric procedure may be applied when the data being analyzed consist merely of rankings or classifications. Nonparametric tests also have several disadvantages. If the assumptions about the underlying distribution are satisfied, then a nonparametric test is less powerful than a parametric test (e.g., t-tests for comparing two sample means). This is due to the fact that potentially useful information is ignored when using nonparametric methods. For instance, the probability of type II error in a nonparametric test, β, would be larger than that of a parametric test. To make β the same, a larger sample size is required for the nonparametric test. Thus, it can be concluded that if the assumptions about the underlying distribution are satisfied, then parametric tests are the best tool; if not, nonparametric tests are more appropriate.

There are many nonparametric tests, but only a few the most efficient and systematic methods will be introduced in this chapter, including rank sum tests, two related samples tests, and two independent samples tests.

10.2 Wilcoxon's Matched Pairs Test

10.2.1 Introduction

When the differences between pairs of observations in a population are normally distributed, a paired t-test can be used to determine the difference. If the assumption of normally distributed differences is not appropriate, the Wilcoxon's matched pairs test can be used instead.

Two or more observations are often gained from the same trial subject, indicating that the populations are related to each other, and not independent from one another. In this case, a test for two related samples is used to evaluate the sample distribution.

The matched pairs signed rank test was proposed by Wilcoxon in 1945, so it is referred to as Wilcoxon's Matched Pairs test. It is often used to evaluate the null hypothesis that the median difference in the underlying populations is equal to 0. If the difference between the two populations is not significant, the sample would have approximately equal numbers of positive and negative ranks. In other words, the median difference is equal to 0, and the distribution is symmetrical. On the other hand, if the numbers of the plus and minus rank sums differ greatly, then the T-value of statistic is very small. The P-value caused by the sampling error is also small, provided that the assumption is right. From Appendix 7, T Distribution (Paired design signed rank test), a certain pattern is apparent—when the n value is certain, the T-value and P-value are directly proportional. As the T-value decreases, the P-value also decreases. The null hypothesis is either rejected or failed to reject at the α level of significance and a conclusion about the test is made.

10.2.2   Method

The steps of conducting a Wilcoxon's Matched Pairs test are demonstrated using the following example.

A sample of 15 patients suffering from asthma participated in an experiment to study the effect of a new treatment on pulmonary function. Among the various measurements recorded were those of forced expiratory volume (liters) in 1 s (FEV_1) before and after application of the treatment. The results were given in Table 10.1. Conduct a test to identify whether the treatment is effective in increasing the FEV_1 level?

Table 10.1 The FEV_1 level before and after the treatment (liters per second)

Patients (1)	Before (2)	After (3)	Difference (4) = (2) − (3)	Rank +(5)	Rank −(6)
1	1.65	1.65	0.00	–	–
2	2.74	2.25	0.49	3	
3	1.02	3.08	−2.06		9
4	1.69	3.37	−1.68		7
5	3.05	3.08	−0.03		1
6	0.92	2.85	−1.93		8
7	1.51	3.70	−2.19		11.5
8	2.76	5.05	−2.29		13
9	2.68	2.36	0.32	2	
10	1.88	4.20	−2.32		14
11	1.83	2.39	−0.56		4
12	1.95	2.98	−1.03		5
13	1.77	3.11	−1.34		6
14	2.51	4.66	−2.15		10
15	2.28	4.47	−2.19		11.5
Sum	–	–	–	5	100

1. Hypothesis
    H_0: There is no significant difference in the FEV$_1$ level, and the median differ-
    ence is 0.
    H_1: There is a significant difference in the FEV$_1$ level, and the median differ-
    ence is not 0.

$$\alpha = 0.05$$

2. Calculate the difference for each pair of observations, as given in the fourth col-
    umn of Table 10.1. Discard any differences of zero so that the sample size is
    reduced by 1 for each pair eliminated. Then, rank the remaining absolute differ-
    ences from smallest to largest. Once the ranks of the absolute differences have
    been determined, give each rank either a plus or minus sign, depending on the
    sign of the difference. Tied differences with opposite signs are assigned the aver-
    age rank. Finally, the complete list of signed ranks, as well as their sum, is given
    in the fifth and sixth columns of Table 10.1.
3. Calculate the T-value. Compute the sum of the positive and negative ranks,
    respectively. The smaller absolute sum is denoted by T, which is shown in the
    fifth and sixth columns. In this example, $T = 5$.
4. Calculate the P-value and make a conclusion.

    (a) Using the appendix: With a sample size of n $\leq$ 25, use the Table 7 in
        Appendix I. If the calculated T-value is larger than the $T_{0.05}$ in the table, con-
        clude that $P > 0.05$; otherwise, $P \leq 0.05$. In the example above, the sample
        size of n was 14, and the T-value was 5. From Appendix I Table 7 T
        Distribution (paired design signed rank test), $T_{0.05} = 21$, $T < T_{0.05} = 21$, $P <$
        0.05; Therefore, the null hypothesis, H_0, at the 0.05 level of significance is
        rejected and it is concluded that the treatment is effective in increasing the
        FEV$_1$ level.
    (b) Approximating a normal distribution: With a sample size of $n > 50$, the
        T-value cannot be found from Table 7 in Appendix I. Since the sum rank T
        is normally distributed approximately, use the normal distribution as follows.

$$\mu_T = n(n+1)/4$$
$$\sigma_T = \sqrt{n(n+1)(2n+1)/24} \tag{10.1}$$

where μ_T is the mean sum of the ranks and σ_T is the standard deviation.
Calculate U using the following formula:

$$U = \frac{|T - \mu_T| - 0.5}{\sigma_T} = \frac{|T - n(n+1)/4| - 0.5}{\sqrt{n(n+1)(2n+1)/24}} \tag{10.2}$$

when many absolute differences have the same value, the U-value will be smaller
than the real one when using Formula 10.2. In this case, calculate the U-value using
Formula 10.3.

$$u = \frac{\left|T - n(n+1)/4\right| - 0.5}{\sqrt{\dfrac{n(n+1)(2n+1)}{24} - \dfrac{\sum\left(t^3_j - t_j\right)}{48}}} \tag{10.3}$$

where t_j is the number of the same absolute differences. For example, when there are two differences of the same value 4, five differences of 6, and three differences of 7, they can be denoted as $t_1 = 2$, $t_2 = 5$, $t_3 = 3$. $\sum(t^3_j - t_j) = (2^3 - 2) \times (5^3 - 5) + (3^3 - 3) = 150$.

Once the U-value is obtained, check Appendix I Table 1 Normal Distribution to get the P-value.

10.2.3 Application of Software

1. The variables (at least two) were defined and the data were inputted into SPSS (as shown in Fig. 10.1).
2. Main output results

From Fig. 10.2, the descriptive statistics of the test (means, deviations, the minimum and maximum of two variables) are shown.

From the information in Fig. 10.3, the mean ranks of the negative and positive are 2.50 and 8.33, and the sums of the ranks are 5.00 and 100.00.

From Fig. 10.4, the Z-value is −2.983 and P-value is 0.003.

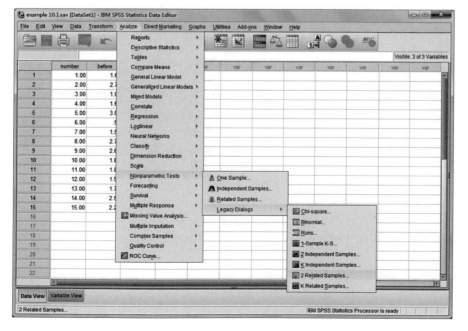

Fig. 10.1 SPSS file

Fig. 10.2 Descriptive
statistics

	N	Mean	Std. Deviation	Minimum	Maximum
before	15	2.0160	.63858	.92	3.05
after	15	3.2800	.97191	1.65	5.05

Ranks

		N	Mean Rank	Sum of Ranks
after - before	Negative Ranks	2[a]	2.50	5.00
	Positive Ranks	12[b]	8.33	100.00
	Ties	1[c]		
	Total	15		

a. after < before

b. after > before

c. after = before

Fig. 10.3 Ranks of variables

Fig. 10.4 Test statistics

Test Statistics[a]

	after - before
Z	-2.983[b]
Asymp. Sig. (2-tailed)	.003

a. Wilcoxon Signed Ranks Test

b. Based on negative ranks.

3. Conclusion

Since the statistics P-value is 0.003 and smaller than 0.05, thus the null hypothesis is rejected. It can then be concluded that there is a significant difference between the FEV_1 level before and after the treatment.

10.3 Tests of Differences Between Two Groups

10.3.1 Introduction

Rank sum tests can also be used to determine the difference of two independent samples. It is more widely used than Wilcoxon's Matched Pairs test when determining the distributions of two populations.

Assume that there are two samples with sample sizes n_1 and n_2 respectively, which come from the same population or two identical populations. The data are randomly divided into group one or group two. The T-value of the sample of size n_1 is the same as or approximately the mean rank value, $n_1(N+1)/2$. If it is not the same, then it is out of the test range (as shown in Appendix I Table 8, T distribution (Wilcoxon Mann–Whitney test, smaller T-value) indicating that the probability of the sample statistic T-value being the described one is small. Therefore, the null hypothesis is rejected; otherwise, the null hypothesis would not be rejected.

10.3.2 Method

Using the information given in Table 10.2, the process of performing a rank sum test is demonstrated.

The level of mental health scores of two group junior high boys are given in Table 10.2. One group comes from a rural junior high school and the other from an urban junior high school. Conduct a test to determine whether there is a significant difference in the level of mental health scores between the two groups.

1. Hypothesis.
   H_0: The distributions of the two group boys are the same.
   H_1: The distributions of the two group boys are not the same.

$$\alpha = 0.05$$

Table 10.2 The level of mental health scores of two group junior high boys

Urban school boys group		Rural school boys group	
Mental health scores	Rank	Mental health scores	Rank
36	15.5	29	11
25	4	50	27
28	10	44	21.5
22	2	26	6
26	6	45	23.5
34	14	48	25.5
27	8.5	41	19.5
21	1	33	13
26	6	51	28
27	8.5	37	17
45	23.5	36	15.5
48	25.5	32	12
39	18		
24	3		
44	21.5		
41	19.5		
$n_1 = 16$	$T = 186.5$	$n_2 = 12$	$T = 219.5$

2. Rank the values of the two groups from the smallest to the largest. The same values in different groups are assigned an average rank. For example, a value of 36 exists both in group urban and group rural. As a result, they are given the average value $[(15 + 16)/2 = 15.5]$.
3. Calculate the T-value. When the sample sizes are different, take the rank sum that is from smaller sample size. When they are the same, take either of the two rank sums. In this example, $n_1 = 16$, $n_2 = 12$, $T = 219.5$
4. Calculate the **P**-value and make a conclusion

(a) Using the Appendix I Table 8 T Distribution (Wilcoxon Mann–Whitney test, smaller T-value), $n_1 \leq 20$, $n_2\text{-}n_1 \leq 10$, of the values of T, compare the smaller value to the values in Table 8. If the values of T is smaller than the $T_{0.05}$ in the table, then $P > 0.05$. Otherwise, $P \leq 0.05$. In this example, the sample size $n_1 = 16$, $n_2 = 12$, the T-value is 219.5. The information from Table 8 indicates that $T_{0.05} = 131$. Since $T = 219.5 > 131$, $P < 0.05$. Therefore, the null hypothesis H_0 at the 0.05 level of significance is rejected, and it can be concluded that the distributions of the two group boys are not the same. The level of mental health scores of urban high school boys is larger than ones of rural high school boys.

(b) Approximating a normal distribution: When the sample size n_1 or $n_2\text{-}n_1$ is outside the test range, U-test is used. In other words, when the sample size is larger, the rank sum approximately follows a normal distribution, so the following equations are applied.

$$\mu_T = n_1 (n+1)/2$$
$$\sigma_T^2 = \frac{n_1 n_2 (n+1)}{12}\left[1 - \frac{\Sigma(t_k^3 - t_k)}{n^3 - n}\right] \tag{10.4}$$

where μ_T is the mean sum of the ranks and σ_T is the standard deviation. Then U can be calculated using the following formula:

$$U = \frac{|T - n_1(n+1)/2| - 0.5}{\sqrt{\sigma_T^2}} \tag{10.5}$$

Once the U-value is obtained, check Appendix I Table 1 for the P-value.

10.3.3 Application of Software

1. The Variables were defined, and the data were input into SPSS.
2. Main output results
   From the information shown in Fig. 10.5, the means, deviations, and the minimum and maximum of the two variables can be found.

	N	Mean	Std. Deviation	Minimum	Maximum
scores	28	35.1786	9.28979	21.00	51.00
group	28	1.4286	.50395	1.00	2.00

Fig. 10.5 Descriptive statistics

Ranks

	group	N	Mean Rank	Sum of Ranks
	urban school boys	16	11.66	186.50
scores	rural school boys	12	18.29	219.50
	Total	28		

Fig. 10.6 Ranks of the variables

Fig. 10.7 Test statistics

Test Statistics[a]

	scores
Mann-Whitney U	50.500
Wilcoxon W	186.500
Z	-2.115
Asymp. Sig. (2-tailed)	.034
Exact Sig. [2*(1-tailed Sig.)]	.033[b]

a. Grouping Variable: group

b. Not corrected for ties.

The information shown in Fig. 10.6 indicates that Group 1 contains 16 samples and Group 2 contains 12. The sums of the ranks are 186.50 and 219.50, respectively.

Using the information shown in Fig. 10.7, the U-value and Z-value, 50.500 and −2.115, respectively, can be obtained. The P-value is 0.033.

3. Conclusion

Since the P-value is 0.033, and smaller than 0.05, thus the null hypothesis is rejected, and it can be concluded that there is a significant difference between the scores levels of urban and rural high school boys.

10.4   Tests of Differences Between K Groups (Independent Samples)

10.4.1   Introduction

The two independent tests mentioned above are the most basic methods. When several samples that are completely random must be tested, the Kruskal–Wallis method, or the H test, is often used. The rank sum of the samples can then be used to test whether the distributions of the populations are the same.

10.4.2   Method

The information given in Table 10.3 is used as an example to show the steps of testing the differences between k group independent samples.

The net book value of equipment capital per bed by hospital type are given in Table 10.3. Conduct a test to determine whether there is a significant difference in the average net book value of equipment capital per bed differs among the three types of hospitals.

1. Hypothesis

    H_0: There is no significant difference in the average net book value of equipment capital per bed among the three types of hospitals or the distributions are the same.

    H_1: There is a significant difference in the average net book value of equipment capital per bed among the three types of hospitals or the distributions are not all the same.

$$\alpha = 0.05$$

2. Rank all the data in the three groups from the smallest to the largest. Data of the same values are assigned the average rank. In this example, there are two values of 1755 in the third and fifth columns, and there are two values of 2650 in the first and fifth columns. Therefore, they are each given the average rank, which is

Table 10.3 The net book value of equipment per bed by hospital type ($)

A		B		C	
Net book value (1)	Rank (2)	Net book value (3)	Rank (4)	Net book value (5)	Rank (6)
2650	6.5	1755	2.5	2785	10
3455	13	2550	5	1755	2.5
3280	11	2425	4	2650	6.5
3355	12	1655	1	3550	14
3680	15	2735	8	2745	9
R_i	57.5		20.5		42
n_i	5		5		5

(2+3)/2 = 2.5, (6+7)/2 = 6.5, respectively. Finally, add the ranks of each group and obtain the rank sum R_i.
3. Calculate the H-value using the following formula:

$$H = \frac{12}{N(N-1)} \sum \frac{R_i^2}{n_i} - 3(N+1) \qquad (10.6)$$

where n_i is the amount of data in each group.
$N = \sum n_i$ is the amount of total data in the three groups.
In this example,

$$H = \frac{12}{15(15+1)} \left(\frac{57.5^2}{5} + \frac{20.5^2}{5} + \frac{42^2}{5} \right) - 3(15+1) = 6.93 \qquad (10.7)$$

When the amount of the same ranks is more than 25% of the whole, the calculated H-value is smaller than the real value, so a correction formula is necessary. The correction formula is as follows:

$$H_c = H / C$$

$$C = 1 - \sum \left(t_j^3 - t_j \right) / \left(N^3 - N \right) \qquad (10.8)$$

4. Calculate the **P**-value and make a conclusion.

With group number $K = 3$ and sample size of $n \leq 5$ in each group, Appendix I Table 9 H Distribution (Kruskal–Wallis H test), can be used to find the P-value. If calculated H-value is larger than $H_{0.05}$ in the table, $P < 0.05$; otherwise, $P > 0.05$. If the smallest sample size is $n \geq 5$, the H-value cannot be found from using Appendix I, Table 9 H distribution. Since the H-value approximately follows the chi-square distribution of $v = k - 1$, the chi-square distribution table (Table 6) can be used to obtain the P-value.

In this example, the group number $K = 3$ and sample size of $n = 5$ in each group. Search the Appendix I Table 9 H distribution (Kruskal-Wallis H test) table on the condition that $H_{0.05} = 5.78$ and $P < 0.05$. In this case, reject the null hypothesis H_0 at the 0.05 level of significance and conclude that there is a significant difference in the average net book value of equipment capital per bed among the three types of hospitals.

10.4.3 Application of Software

1. Variables were defined and the data were inputted into SPSS (as shown in Fig. 10.9).
2. Main output results
    From Fig. 10.8, the descriptive statistics of the test (e.g., means, deviations, the minimum and maximum of two variables) can be obtained.

	N	Mean	Std. Deviation	Minimum	Maximum
dollar	15	2735.00	654.198	1655	3680
group	15	2.0000	.84515	1.00	3.00

Fig. 10.8 Descriptive statistics

Fig. 10.9 Ranks of variables

Ranks

group		N	Mean Rank
dollar	1.00	5	11.50
	2.00	5	4.10
	3.00	5	8.40
	Total	15	

Fig. 10.10 Test statistics

Test Statistics[a,b]

	dollar
Chi-Square	6.930
df	2
Asymp. Sig.	.031

a. Kruskal Wallis Test

b. Grouping Variable: group

The information in Fig. 10.9 shows that each group contains five samples and that their mean ranks are different from one another. The mean rank of Group 1 is 11.50; Group 2, 4.10; Group 3, 8.40.

The information in Fig. 10.10 shows the K-W statistic (6.930) and the P-value (0.031).

3. Conclusion

Since the P-value is smaller than 0.05, the null hypothesis is rejected, and it can be concluded that there is a significant difference in the average net book value of equipment capital per bed among the three types of hospitals.

10.5 Tests of Differences Between K Groups (Nominal Explanatory and Ordinal Variable)

10.5.1 Introduction

The k independent tests mentioned above represent the most basic methods. When several samples (two or k groups) that are nominal and an ordinal response variable, we can use an extension of the Wilcoxon Rank Sum test that was described. This involves ranking the subjects from smallest to largest in terms of the measurement of interest (there will be many ties), and compute the rank-sum for each level of the nominal explanatory variable. We then compare the mean ranks among the k groups by the Kruskal-Wallis test.

10.5.2 Method

The information given in Table 10.4 is used as an example to show the steps of testing the differences between nominal explanatory and ordinal variables.

A study was conducted to compare three types of antibiotics in patients with lower respiratory tract infection. The outcomes are given in Table 10.4. Conduct a test to determine whether there is a significant difference in the average cure effect of among the three types of antibiotics.

1. Hypothesis

   H_0: There is no significant difference in the cure effect of among the three types of antibiotics.

   H_1: There is a significant difference in the cure effect of among the three types of antibiotics.

$$\alpha = 0.05$$

Table 10.4 The cure effect of among the three types of antibiotics

Therapeutic outcome	Drug types				Rank range	Mean rank	Rank sum		
	A	B	C	Total			A	B	C
Cure	9	12	10	31	1–31	16	144	192	160
Partial cure	12	18	16	46	32–77	54.5	654	981	872
Antibiotic extended	15	22	32	69	78–146	112	1680	2464	3584
Antibiotic changed	69	68	54	191	147–337	242	16,698	16,456	13,068
Death	75	65	70	210	338–547	442.5	33,187.5	28,762.5	30,975
Total	180	185	182	547	–	–	52,363.5	48,855.5	48,659

2. Rank all the data in the three groups from the smallest to the largest. Data of the same values are assigned the average rank. In this example, there are five ordinal levels which are same values in the fifth column. Therefore, they are each given the average rank, for example, the 'Cure' level, which is $(1+31)/2 = 16$, the rank sum of A group is $16 \times 9 = 144$, next B group and C group are $12 \times 16 = 192$ and $10 \times 16 = 160$, respectively. The rest levels can be done in the same manner. Finally, add the ranks of each group and obtain the total rank sum.
3. Calculate the H-value using the following formula:

$$H = \frac{12}{547(547+1)} \left(\frac{52363.5^2}{180} + \frac{48855.5^2}{185} + \frac{48659^2}{182} \right) - 3(547+1) = 3.11$$

In this example the amount of the same ranks is more than 25% of the whole; the calculated H-value is smaller than the real value, so a correction H-value is necessary.

$$C = 1 - \Sigma\left(t_j^3 - t_j\right) / \left(N^3 - N\right)$$

$$C = 1 - \Sigma\left[\left(31^3 - 31\right) + \left(46^3 - 46\right) + \left(69^3 - 69\right) + \left(191^3 - 191\right) + \left(210^3 - 210\right)\right]$$
$$/ \left(547^3 - 547\right) = 0.898$$

$$H_C = H / C = 3.11 / 0.898 = 3.463$$

4. Calculate the P-value and make a conclusion.

With group number $K = 3$ and sample size of $n \leq 5$ in each group, Appendix I Table 9, H Distribution (Kruskal–Wallis H test), can be used to find the P-value. If calculated H-value is larger than $H_{0.05}$ in the table, $P < 0.05$; otherwise, $P > 0.05$.

If the smallest sample size is $n \geq 5$, the H-value cannot be found from using Appendix 10.4. Since the H-value approximately follows the chi-square distribution of $v = k - 1$, the chi-square distribution table can be used to obtain the P-value.

In this example, the group number $K = 3$ and sample size of n ≥ 5 in each group indicates that Appendix I, Table 9 H Distribution cannot be used. Search the Chi-square distribution table (Table 6) on the condition that $v = 3-1 = 2$. $\chi^2_{0.05(2)} = 5.99$ and $P > 0.05$. In this case, not reject the null hypothesis H_0 at the 0.05 level of significance and conclude that there is no significant difference in the cure effect of among the three types of antibiotics.

10.5.3   Application of Software

1. Variables were defined and the data were inputted into SPSS.
2. Main output results

	N	Mean	Std. Deviation	Minimum	Maximum
outcome	547	3.9196	1.16297	1.00	5.00
group	547	2.0037	.81424	1.00	3.00

Fig. 10.11 Descriptive statistics

Fig. 10.12 Ranks of variables

Ranks

group		N	Mean Rank
outcome	A	180	290.91
	B	185	264.08
	C	182	267.36
	Total	547	

Fig. 10.13 Test statistics

Test Statistics[a,b]

	outcome
Chi-Square	3.463
df	2
Asymp. Sig.	.177

a. Kruskal Wallis Test

b. Grouping Variable: group

From Fig. 10.11, the descriptive statistics of the test (e.g., means, deviations, the minimum and maximum of two variables) can be obtained.

The information in Fig. 10.12 shows that each group contains different samples and that their mean ranks are different from one another. The mean rank of Group 1 is 290.91; Group 2, 264.08; Group 3, 267.36.

The information in Fig. 10.13 shows the Chi-Square statistic (3.463) and the P-value (0.177).

3. Conclusion

Since the P-value is larger than 0.05, the null hypothesis is not rejected, and it can be concluded that there is no significant difference in the cure effect of among the three types of antibiotics.

Chapter Summary

1. Since nonparametric tests are free from the population parameters, they are also known as distribution-free tests.

2. Nonparametric tests can be used in the following cases: the underlying distribution is unknown; the population is not normally distributed; the data are described as levels, grades, or sequences; the population parameters, such as the homogeneity of variances, don't meet all of the requirements for testing; some data are too large or uncertain.
3. It is better to use parametric tests when all of the testing requirements are fulfilled. If not, nonparametric tests are an efficient test method. However, if the assumptions underlying a parametric test are satisfied, the nonparametric method is less powerful. Since some information is missed in nonparametric statistics, the probability of an error type II is higher than that of parametric statistics.
4. The main points and details of the three test methods in this chapter are summarized in the following table (Table 10.5).

Table 10.5 Main points and details of the three test methods

Test method	Main points	Details
Two related samples test	1. Rank the absolute difference from the smallest to the largest. Give either a plus or a minus sign. Search the appendix to get the boundary value of T. If T is within the range, $P > \alpha$; otherwise, $P \leq \alpha$ 2. If n > 50, a U-test is more appropriate	1. Tied differences of opposite signs are assigned the average rank 2. Discard any differences of zero 3. If $n < 5$, no valuable conclusion can be made
Two independent samples test	1. Rank the data of the two groups from the smallest to the largest. Denote the smaller n as T and search the appendix to get the boundary value. If T is within the range, $P > \alpha$; otherwise, $P \leq \alpha$ 2. If n > 20 or n_1-n_2 > 10, a U-test is more appropriate	1. Tied data which are in different groups are assigned the average rank. 2. If many ranks are the same, the correction formula should be used instead.
K-Independent-samples test	1. Rank the data of K groups from the smallest to the larges, and calculate the rank sum T 2. Calculate the H-value and search the statistical table to get the boundary value; If $N > 15$ or $n > 5$, refer to the appendix of χ^2 by $v = k - 1$, and get the P-value 3. If there was significant difference among groups, rank sum test between any two groups should be done	1. Tied data which are in different groups are assigned the average rank 2. If many ranks are the same, the correction formula should be used instead

Chapter 11
Correlation and Simple Linear Regression

Liqin Wang, Ying Guan, and Xia Li

Objectives
Simple correlation and regression analysis are used to determine whether a relationship exists between two variables. Pearson's correlation coefficient is used for measuring linear relationships and Spearman's rank correlation coefficient for ranked relationships between two continuous variables. When estimating the linear relationship between a predictor and an outcome variable, a simple linear regression analysis is conducted. The purpose of this chapter is to answer these questions statistically: (1) Are two variables linear related? If so, what type of relationship exists? What is the strength of the relationship? (2) How to estimate the linear dependency relation between the predictor and response variable by the simple linear regression equation? SPSS software is used to measure the correlation coefficient and establish a simple linear regression model form the example.

Key Concepts
Pearson's correlation coefficient; Spearman's rank correlation coefficient; Simple linear regression

L. Wang (✉)
School of Public Health, Hebei Medical University, Shijiazhuang, China
e-mail: wliqin673696@163.co

Y. Guan
School of Public Health, Southern Medical University, Guangzhou, China

X. Li
Department of Mathematics and Statistics, La Trobe University, Melbourne, VIC, Australia

© Zhengzhou University Press 2024
X. Guo, F. Xue (eds.), *Textbook of Medical Statistics*,
https://doi.org/10.1007/978-981-99-7390-3_11

157

11.1   Introduction

The purpose of a correlation analysis is to measure and interpret the strength of a linear or nonlinear relationship (e.g., exponential, polynomial, and logistic) between two continuous variables. When conducting a correlation analysis, the term "association" is used to refer to "linear association." This chapter focuses on Pearson's and Spearman's correlation coefficients. Both correlation coefficients take on values between -1 and $+1$, ranging from negative correlations (-1) to no correlations (0) to positive correlations $(+1)$. The sign of the correlation coefficient defines the direction of the relationship. The absolute value of the correlation coefficient indicates the strength of the correlation. The linear (i.e., Pearson) and rank (i.e., Spearman) coefficients are commonly used for measuring linear and general relationships between two variables.

As a statistical tool, a regression analysis investigates relationship in variables. Statisticians often wish to predict, or explain, one variable in terms of others. Regression modeling can help solve this problem. The aim of this chapter is to introduce the simplest type of regression model, in which both the response variable and the single predictor are measured using numerical scales. In a simple linear regression, there are two variables: an independent variable, also called an explanatory variable (X), and a dependent variable, also called a response variable (Y). If both X and Y are known, the best straight line through the data is desired.

The regression method was first used to examine the relationship between the heights of fathers and the heights of sons. The two variables were related, but the slope was less than 1. The result indicated that a tall father tended to have sons shorter than him, and a short father tended to have sons taller than him. The term "regression" is now used for many types of curve-fitting situations.

In general, the goal of linear regressions is to find the best line that predicts Y by X. A linear regression does this by finding the line that minimizes the sum of the squares of the vertical distances of the points from the line. That is, the stronger the relationship is between variables, the more accurate the prediction is.

11.2   Correlation Analysis

Correlation is a measure of association between two variables that are not designated as either dependent or independent. This chapter investigates the relationships between two quantitative variables. The two most popular correlation coefficients are Pearson's correlation coefficient and Spearman's correlation coefficient. When calculating a correlation coefficient for ordinal data, Spearman's technique is preferred. For interval or ratio-type data, Pearson's technique is performed.

The value of a correlation coefficient varies from -1 to $+1$; -1 indicates a perfect negative correlation; while $+1$ indicates a perfect positive correlation. A correlation of zero means there is no linear relationship between the two variables. If two variables have a negative correlation, the value of one variable increases as the value of the other variable decreases, or vice versa. In other words, the variables are inversely related. There is a positive correlation between the two variables, the values of both variables travel in the same direction (i.e., the two variables are directly related). To summarize the main components of correlations:

- The correlation value is between −1 and +1.
- A correlation measures the degree of linear association between the two variables.
- If the correlation coefficient is equal to +1, there is a perfect positive association between the two variables.
- If the correlation coefficient is equal to −1, there is a perfect negative association between the two variables.
- If the correlation coefficient is equal to 0, there is no linear association between the two variables.
- The correlation is invariant to the linear change of the scale for the variables.
- A positive correlation indicates that if X is larger than its average, then the corresponding Y is more likely to be larger than its average as well.
- A negative correlation indicates that if X is larger than its average, then the corresponding Y is more likely to be smaller than its average.

11.2.1   Scatter Plots

A scatter plot is a useful summary for a set of bivariate data (i.e., two variables), usually created before a linear correlation coefficient or regression line are fitted to the data. A scatter plot is a visual way to describe the relationship between the independent and dependent variables. A scatter plot is often used to identify potential associations between two variables (e.g., X and Y). A **positive association** between these two variables would be indicated on a scatter plot by an upward trend (positive slope), where a bigger X corresponds to a bigger Y and a smaller X corresponds to a smaller Y. A **negative association** would be indicated by the opposite effect (i.e., negative slope), where a bigger X corresponds to a smaller Y. There also may not be any notable association, for which a scatter plot would not indicate any trends whatsoever. The following plots demonstrate the appearance of positively associated (a), negatively associated (b), and non-associated variables (c) (Fig. 11.1).

11.2.2   Pearson's Correlation Coefficient

Statisticians use a statistic called the correlation coefficient to represent the strength of the linear relationship between two quantitative variables. The symbol for the sample correlation coefficient is r. The symbol for the population correlation coefficient is ρ (rho). The Pearson correlation coefficient is referred to the sample

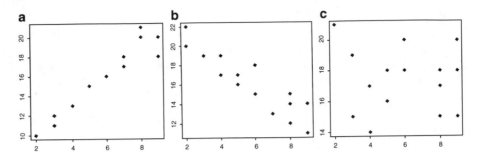

Fig. 11.1 Scatter plot of relationships

correlation coefficient (r), product-moment correlation coefficient, or coefficient of correlation. It was introduced by Galton in 1877 and later developed by Pearson. It measures the linear relationship between two random variables. For example, when the value of the predictor is manipulated (i.e., increased or decreased) by a fixed amount, the outcome changes proportionally (linearly). A linear correlation coefficient can be computed by means of the data and the sample means. When a scientific study is planned, the required sample size may be computed on the basis of a certain hypothesized value with the desired statistical power at a specified level of significance. A Pearson correlation is often followed by a P value that tests whether there is a linear association or no linear association (if $r = 0$). This P value is only useful when the variables are normally distributed. In other words, both variables are approximately normally distributed and their joint distribution is bivariate normal distribution.

Pearson's formula for calculating the correlation coefficient, r, is as follows:

$$
\begin{aligned}
r &= \frac{l_{xy}}{\sqrt{l_{xx}l_{yy}}} = \frac{\sum_{i=1}^{n}(x_i - \bar{x})(y_i - \bar{y})}{\sqrt{\sum_{i-1}^{n}(x_i - \bar{x})^2 (y_i - \bar{y})^2}} \\[2mm]
l_{xx} &= \sum_{i=1}^{n} x_i^2 - \frac{1}{n}\left(\sum_{i=1}^{n} x_i\right)^2 \\[2mm]
l_{yy} &= \sum_{i=1}^{n} y_i^2 - \frac{1}{n}\left(\sum_{i=1}^{n} y_i\right)^2 \\[2mm]
l_{xy} &= \sum_{i=1}^{n} x_i y_i - \frac{1}{n}\left(\sum_{i=1}^{n} x_i\right)\left(\sum_{i=1}^{n} y_i\right) \\[2mm]
\text{or } r &= \frac{XY - \overline{XY}}{SD_X * SD_Y}
\end{aligned}
\tag{11.1}
$$

where N represents the number of pairs of data, Σ denotes the summation of the items indicated, $\overline{XY}$ is the mean of all $X*Y$ values, SD_X is the standard deviation of X, SD_Y is the standard deviation of Y.

When you get the sample correlation coefficient, the next step is to test if there is any correlation in the population level. Is there any correlation in population level, or is the sample correlation just normal sample variability? What is the estimated correlation coefficient of the population? These questions can be answered by inferential statistics. In particular, a hypothesis test can be conducted to test whether there is a linear relationship between the two variables. In order to perform a hypothesis test, a null hypothesis must be set up as

$H_0 : \rho = 0$ (there is no linear correlation in the population and no linear relationship between X and Y).

If H_0 is true, then the correlation coefficient (r) of the sample is within normal sample variability for a sample of this size drawn from a population where $\rho = 0$. If H_0 is false, then the alternative hypothesis (H_1) is accepted, implying that there is a linear relationship between variables X and Y in the population (H_1: $\rho \neq 0$). The distribution of the sample statistics must be known in order to determine whether to accept or reject the null hypothesis. Assuming that the true population correlation ρ is 0, and then the correlations of the sample generates a statistic that follows the student's t-distribution:

$$t = r \cdot \sqrt{\frac{n-2}{1-r^2}} \quad \text{With} \quad df = n-2 \qquad (11.2)$$

From the t statistic, the P value can be computed. This P value indicates how likely it is that the sample r was obtained by chance if there was no correlation in the population. If the P value is very small (usually chosen at a threshold of 0.05), H_0 is rejected, and it can be concluded that the correlation of sample is not due to chance, and there is a correlation in population.

11.2.3   Spearman's Rank Correlation Coefficient

If the data do not follow a normal distribution, or if outliers are present, the correlation of the ranks of the X values and the Y values should be computed. Such a correlation is known as a Spearman correlation. A Spearman correlation is robust for non-normal distributions and outliers, and the associated P value is therefore more generally applicable. When the data are organized in ranks, the Spearman correlation for ranked data (Spearman ρ) can be computed and significance can be tested like the Pearson correlation coefficient r. The Spearman ρ measures the linear association between pairs of ranks. If the data are not organized into ranks, the raw data can be converted into ranks prior to computing the correlation coefficient. The Spearman coefficient measures the degree of the monotonic relationship between the original variables. If Y increases by each time X increases (i.e., the slope of the line relating X to Y is always positive), then there is a perfect positive monotonic relationship. However, it is not necessarily a perfect linear relationship (for which the slope must be constant). Spearman's formula for calculating the correlation coefficient, r, is as follows:

$$r_S = 1 - \frac{6 \times \sum d^2}{n(n^2 - 1)} \tag{11.3}$$

where r_s is the Spearman rank correlation coefficient, d is the difference between the ranks of each pair of corresponding values of the variables X and Y, n is the number of pairs of values in the sample.

The value of the Spearman correlation coefficient always varies between -1 and $+1$ as a pure number without units or dimensions. When using such coefficient, there are two sets of ranks assigned to the variables X and Y. The original observations may either be in ranks or in numerical values ranked by magnitude. In addition to interpreting the magnitude and direction of a correlation coefficient, the significance of sample correlation must be tested. The null hypothesis states that no correlation exists and that whatever value of correlation between the two examined variables is due to sampling error.

As the data (i.e., the ranks) used in the Spearman test are not drawn from a bivariate normal population, the tables of critical values have different values. If the sample size is smaller than 50, the Spearman critical values table can be used. If the sample size is larger than 50, the correlation of samples r_s follows a student's t-distribution:

$$t_{r_s} = r_s \cdot \sqrt{\frac{n-2}{1-r_s^2}} \quad \text{With} \quad df = n - 2. \tag{11.4}$$

The P value can then be computed. If the P value is very small (usually chosen at a threshold of 0.05), H_0 should be rejected, and it can be concluded that the sample correlation is not due to chance, so there is a correlation in population.

11.3   Application of Correlation Analysis

Example 11.1 A medical center collected the weight and height data of some children in Beijing, 20 of which are used in the correlation analysis below (Table 11.1).

Here, Height is X and Weight is Y. Do these two variables have a linear relationship?

Table 11.1 The weight and height data of 20 children

ID	Height (cm)	Weight (kg)
1	89.0	11.7
2	88.8	11.8
3	90.9	12.0
4	87.4	12.2
5	88.7	12.4
6	90.8	12.5
7	92.5	12.6
8	92.2	12.7
9	88.4	12.8
10	94.0	13.0
11	92.1	13.1
12	90.5	13.2
13	89.8	13.3
14	94.1	13.4
15	89.2	13.5
16	92.4	13.6
17	95.1	13.7
18	90.7	13.8
19	93.9	14.0
20	93.8	14.4

11.3.1 Build a SPSS Data File

In the first, we quantify the quantitative variables, Height and Weight.

The process of inputting the data into SPSS is File → Open → Data → select the data location or copy the text data file into SPSS. Then, we can determine the data type and the number of decimal places.

11.3.2 Pearson's Correlation by SPSS

The main process to show the correlate between Y and X by SPSS 20.0 is

Analyze → Correlate → Bivariate → X, Y → select to Variables → correlation coefficients → OK.

Step by step process:

1. Using SPSS software, Graph → Scatter/dot… → Select Simple Scatter → Define (Fig. 11.2)
2. Select Weight (kg) to the Y-Axis and Height (cm) to the X-Axis → OK.

Fig. 11.2 Using SPSS to create a scatter plot

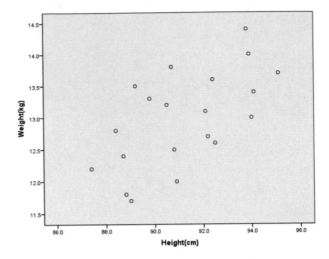

Fig. 11.3 Bivariate correlations dialog box

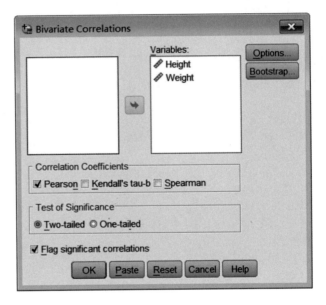

3. Analyze → Correlate → Bivariate, we select the Height and Weight to Variables as shown in Fig. 11.3 bivariate correlations dialog box, select Pearson (if ordinal data select Spearman), then click on OK.

11.3.3 Main output results

Figure 11.4 correlations shows the Pearson Correlation between Height and Weight. The figure showed that Pearson Correlation $r = 0.611$, $P = 0.004$. There is a significant correlation relationship between the weight and height of Children in Beijing.

Fig. 11.4 Pearson
correlation result

Correlations

		Height	Weight
Height	Pearson Correlation	1	.611**
	Sig. (2-tailed)		.004
	N	20	20
Weight	Pearson Correlation	.611**	1
	Sig. (2-tailed)	.004	
	N	20	20

**. Correlation is significant at the 0.01 level (2-tailed).

11.4 Simple Linear Regression

11.4.1 Introduction to Simple Linear Regression

The equation of the regression, which represents the line of best fit, describes how the response variable varies with only one predictor. If Y is a linear function of X, then $Y = \alpha + \beta X$, which is a straight line when graphed. When $X = 0$, $Y = \alpha$, α is known as the intercept. The coefficient b of X represents the amount of change in Y corresponding to one unit of change in X. This is the slope of the line. To understand the basic concepts of a regression analysis, consider the following simple linear regression model for investigating a relationship of a response variable Y and a predictor X.

$$Y = \alpha + \beta X + \varepsilon \qquad (11.5)$$

The random error ε is assumed to be normally distributed with a mean of 0 and variance σ^2. This assumption implies that Y is also normally distributed with $\mu_y = \alpha + \beta X$ and $\sigma^y{}_2 = \sigma^2$. In this model, α, β, and σ^2 are unknown and must be estimated. If $\beta = 0$, then X is not a significant predictor of Y. If $\sigma^2 = 0$, then there is a perfect linear relationship between Y and X, and the parameters β and α can be estimated using just two observations of pairs (Y, X). The followings are assumptions of a simple linear regression between a dependent (response) variable Y and the independent variable X:

- Linearity: the average value of the dependent variable has a straight line relationship with the independent variable
- Independence: the observations are randomly and independently selected
- Normality: the values of the dependent variable are normally distributed for observations with the same value of the independent variable

- Equal variation: the variation in the values of the dependent variable is equal for observations with the same value of the independent variable, regardless of the value of the independent variable

11.4.2 Estimating the Regression Coefficient and Hypothesis Testing

The least squared (LS) method is usually used to estimate the regression coefficients. Minimizing the squared differences between the line and the actual values of Y creates an estimate close to all values of Y. The basic principle of the LS method is to look for the best regression coefficients that minimize the residual sum of the squares (RSS) between the observed value Y_i and the estimated value $Y_{i}^{'}$. The estimated values of the regression coefficients by the LS method just meet the BLUE (best linear unbiased estimator) principle.

$$b = \frac{l_{XY}}{l_{XX}}$$

$$a = \overline{Y} - b\overline{X}$$

(11.6)

A t-test is used to test whether the overall regression coefficient is zero. The hypotheses of the test are

$$H_0 : \beta = 0$$

$$H_1 : \beta \neq 0$$

$$\alpha = 0.05.$$

The t-test statistic is

$$t_b = \frac{b}{S_b} \quad \text{With} \quad df = n - 2$$

(11.7)

$$S_b = \frac{S_{YX}}{\sqrt{l_{XX}}} \quad S_{YX} = \sqrt{\frac{SS_E}{n-2}}$$

where S_b is the standard error of the regression coefficient. b is the regression coefficient.

The t-test is used to conduct hypothesis tests on the regression coefficients obtained in simple linear regressions. The test indicates whether the fitted regression model adequately explains variations in the observations or if there is no true relationship between X and Y. If the desired significance level is 0.1 and the P value is smaller than 0.1, then a relationship exists between X and Y, so the null hypothesis is rejected.

A F-test can also be conducted to test for a linear relationship. The statistic used is based on the F distribution. If the null hypothesis is true, then the statistic:

$$F = \frac{MS_R}{MS_E} = \frac{SS_R/1}{SS_E/(n-2)}$$

$$SS_R = \sum_{i=1}^{n}\left(\hat{y}_i - \bar{y}\right)^2 \qquad (11.8)$$

$$SS_E = \sum_{i=1}^{n}\hat{e}_i^2 = \sum_{i=1}^{n}\left(y_i - \hat{y}_i\right)^2$$

follows the F distribution with 1 degree of freedom in the numerator and $(n-2)$ degrees of freedom in the denominator.

11.4.3 Hypothesis Testing of a Regression Equation

An analysis of variance (ANOVA) is another method of testing for the significance of a regression. This approach uses the variance of the observed data to determine if a regression model can be applied to the observed data. The observed variance is partitioned into components that are then used in a test for significance of regression.

From the results of ANOVA, the coefficient of determination can be calculated to reflect the proficiency of the regression equation. The coefficient of determination is usually written as R^2 and the formula is

$$R^2 = \frac{SS_R}{SS_T}, \quad \text{with}$$

$$SS_R = \sum_{i=1}^{n}\left(\hat{y}_i - \bar{y}\right)^2 \qquad SS_T = \sum_{i=1}^{n}\left(y_i - \bar{y}\right)^2. \qquad (11.9)$$

The estimated model may be perceived to be inadequate unless R^2 is high, say 85 % or more. Low R^2 values suggest the need to investigate additional predictors.

11.5 Application

Example
The data used below are taken from the Pearson correlation example. The data have a linear trend between X and Y.

11.5.1 Build a SPSS Data File

Same to Sect. 11.3.1.

11.5.2 Simple Linear Regression by SPSS

The main process to show the simple linear regression between Y and X by SPSS 20.0 is

Analyze → Regression → Linear → Y → select to Dependent → X select to Independent(s) → Method → Stepwise → Options → OK. Step by step process:

1. Analyze → Regression → Linear, enter Linear Regression model, as shown in Fig. 11.5.
2. In Linear Regression window, we select "Weight" as Dependent Y, "Height" as Independent X, and chooses enter in Methods. In SPSS20.0.
3. Click on statistics. Select estimates, model fit.
4. Click on plots. Select ZRESID as Y-axis, DEPENDNT as X-axis. Click on continue, and then click on OK.

11.5.3 Main Output Results

Figure 11.6 model summary shows the R square in the models. We know from the figure that $R = 0.611$ in model, $R^2 = 0.373$, and standard error of the estimate $= 0.6094$.

Figure 11.7 shows the testing results in the model. $F = 10.723$, $P = 0.004$, when $\alpha = 0.05$. So we can consider there is linear relationship between Y and X.

Fig. 11.5 Linear regression model dialog box

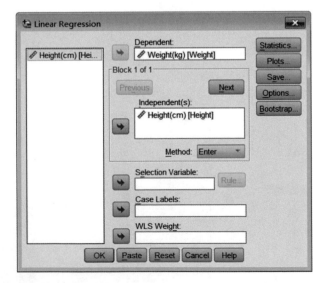

Fig. 11.6 Model summary
for regression

Model Summary[b]

Model	R	R Square	Adjusted R Square	Std. Error of the Estimate
1	.611[a]	.373	.339	.6094

a. Predictors: (Constant), Height(cm)

b. Dependent Variable: Weight(kg)

ANOVA[a]

Model		Sum of Squares	df	Mean Square	F	Sig.
1	Regression	3.982	1	3.982	10.723	.004[b]
	Residual	6.684	18	.371		
	Total	10.666	19			

a. Dependent Variable: Weight

b. Predictors: (Constant), Height

Fig. 11.7 ANVOA table for regression

Coefficients[a]

Model		Unstandardized Coefficients		Standardized Coefficients	t	Sig.
		B	Std. Error	Beta		
1	(Constant)	-5.541	5.659		-.979	.340
	Height	.203	.062	.611	3.275	.004

a. Dependent Variable: Weight

Fig. 11.8 Coefficient show the regression coefficient and the hypothesis testing

We can finally obtain the simple linear regression equation from Fig. 11.8.

$$\hat{Y} = -5.541 + 0.203X$$

11.5.4   Conclusion

Make the decision. Reject the null hypothesis at the 5% level of significance (2-tailed test). There is a significant linear relationship between the weight and height of Children in Beijing.

Chapter Summary
1. Correlations and simple linear regression analyses are very useful. A correlation analysis measures and interprets the strength of linear or rank relationships between two continuous variables.
2. If the data do not appear to be normally distributed or outliers are present, the correlation of the ranks of X values and Y values can be computed in a Spearman correlation.
3. A simple linear regression analysis deals with only one dependent variable and one independent variable. It describes how the dependent variable varies with the values of independent variable.

Chapter 12
Multiple Linear Regression Analysis

Xiuhua Guo, Xiangtong Liu, and Guirong Song

Objectives

Multiple linear regression is the estimation of the linear relationship between a dependent variable and one or more independent variables or covariates. The objective is to give a more detailed description of the regression tool and to touch upon related statistical topics like collinearity and interaction. The SPSS Software was used to establish a multiple linear regression model from the example.

Key Concepts

Multiple linear regression; Linearity; Independency; Partial regression coefficient; Multicollonearity

12.1 Introduction

Linear regression is a statistical method that studies the linear relationship between one dependent variable and one independent variable. However, when we try to solve the practical problems, several indexes (independent variables) may influence the changes of one indicator variable (dependent variable). For instance, the following factors: insulin, glycosylated hemoglobin, serum total cholesterol, triglyceride

X. Guo (✉) · X. Liu
School of Public Health, Capital Medical University, Beijing, China
e-mail: guoxiuh@ccmu.edu.cn

G. Song
School of Public Health, Dalian Medical University, Dalian, China

© Zhengzhou University Press 2024
X. Guo, F. Xue (eds.), *Textbook of Medical Statistics*,
https://doi.org/10.1007/978-981-99-7390-3_12

all affect the changes in diabetic patients' blood sugar; the score of activity of daily living (ADL) of the patients can be impacted by the age, sex, length of hospital stay, the lesion types, the lesion location, the onset to rehabilitation admission's interval, and the impact of baseline ADL. Some practical problems like these need to be analyzed by multiple linear regression to explore the relationship between one dependent variable and several independent variables.

12.2   Introduction to Multiple Linear Regression

Multiple linear regression is a method that studies the relationship between one dependent variable and several independent variables.

12.2.1   Data Structure

If we know that when p variables take different values, they can affect the value of another variable, we call these p variables the independent variables, and call the affected variable the dependent variable. The multiple linear regression can be applied when the dependent variable is an approximate normal distribution of continuous variable, while the independent variables are series of independent numerical variables, binary variables or ordinal variables. Suppose the independent variables are $X_1, \cdots, X_p$, and the dependent variable is Y, the data structure of multiple linear regression can be given in Table 12.1.

12.2.2   Dummy Variable

The independent variables in multiple linear regression can be continuous variables (like age, blood pressure) and binary variables (like sex). The ordinal variables (like the stages of tumor and therapeutic classification) and multinomial variables cannot be applied to the analysis directly. They have to be transformed to several binary

Table 12.1 Data structure of the multiple linear regression

Number	X_1	X_2	...	X_p	Y
1	a_{11}	a_{12}	...	a_{1p}	y_1
2	a_{21}	a_{22}	...	a_{2p}	y_2
...	...	...	...	...	...
n	a_{n1}	a_{n2}	...	a_{np}	y_n

variables before applying in the regression models. We call the process of this transformation is dummying, and the transformed binary variables are called dummy variables. In general, to one ordinal variable or one multinomial variables, the number of the binary variables is equal to the number of the type of ordinal or multinomial variables minus 1.

For instance, blood type is a multinomial variable, which can be classified to four types: A, B, AB, and O. These four types can be described by three binary variables. Suppose type O is the reference variable, then

$$X_1 = \begin{cases} 0 & NotA \\ 1 & A \end{cases} \quad X_2 = \begin{cases} 0 & NotB \\ 1 & B \end{cases} \quad X_3 = \begin{cases} 0 & NotA\,B \\ 1 & AB \end{cases}$$

We can get Table 12.2:

The quantification of the ordinal variables can use multiple dummy variables, just like that on the multinomial variables. We can base on the specific problems to make simple quantification by scoring. For instance, the overall effect of medical evaluation of patients can be divided into very poor, poor, ordinary, good, and very good. The five classifications are valued by 0, 1, 2, 3, and 4. If we know one variable's grade distance is not constant or cannot be measured by the same interval, we cannot assign the same class distance, or its equation to the dependent variable may be distorted.

12.2.3 Prerequisite and Residual Analysis

The prerequisites for multiple linear regression are the same as those for simple linear regression, which require the data to meet criteria for linearity, independence, normal distribution, and equal variance, as summarized by the acronym LINE. **Linearity** is the linear relation between dependent variable Y and a couple of independent variables; **Independency** means that every single individual in a sample is independent with each other; Dependent variable Y must obey **normal distribution** when the values of independent variables are already given; When the independent variables are different, the overall **variance** of the dependent variable (mark σ^2) keeps **equality**.

Table 12.2 Describe blood type by binary dummy variables

Blood type	Variables		
	X_1	X_2	X_3
A	1	0	0
B	0	1	0
AB	0	0	1
O	0	0	0

12.3 Multiple Linear Regression

12.3.1 Multiple Linear Regression Equation

The multiple linear regression equation is an extension of the simple linear regression, and the model is expressed as follows:

$$\hat{Y} = b_0 + b_1 X_1 + b_2 X_2 + \ldots + b_p X_p \tag{12.1}$$

where b_0 is the constant, also called the Y-axis intercept. It is the estimate of the general parameter β_0. b_i is the partial regression coefficient of independent variable Xi and also the estimate of the general parameter β_i. Keeping other independent variables in the equation constant, it shows that since the variable Xi increases (or decrease) one unit, the estimated average change in variable Y is bi units.

In many research studies, we have to evaluate the impact of one single independent variable on the dependent variable. Therefore, we must standardize the independent variables to make them dimensionless units that show the relative changes in variables. Equation (12.2) shows the usual standardized method.

$$X_i' = \frac{X_i - \bar{X}_i}{S_i}. \tag{12.2}$$

12.3.2 Hypothesis Testing of Regression Equation

From the result of ANOVA, we can calculate the coefficient of determination to reflect the proficiency of the regression equation. The coefficient of determination is usually written by R^2, and the formula is

$$R^2 = \frac{SS_{\text{regression}}}{SS_{\text{sum}}}. \tag{12.3}$$

Except the coefficient of determination, we also use the adjusted R^2 (R_{ad}^2). It can be computed as follows:

$$R_{\text{ad}}^2 = 1 - \frac{MS_{\text{residual}}}{MS_{\text{sum}}} = 1 - \frac{SS_{\text{residual}}/(n-p-1)}{SS_{\text{sum}}/(n-1)} = 1 - (1-R^2)\frac{n-1}{n-p-1}. \tag{12.4}$$

12.3.3 Estimate of Regression Coefficient and Hypothesis Testing

Least squared (LS) method is also usually used to estimate the partial regression coefficient in multiple linear regression. The basic principle of LS is to look for the best partial regression coefficients b_0, b_1, b_2, $\cdots$, b_p make the residual sum of square (RSS) between the observed value Y_i and the estimated value $\hat{Y}_i$ minimum. The estimated values of the partial regression coefficients by LS are the ones just meet the LINE principle.

Although the overall partial regression coefficient is zero, we still cannot get sample partial regression coefficient zero because of the sampling error. Therefore, we must run the hypothesis testing on the partial regression coefficients to infer if the overall partial regression coefficient is zero. If the overall partial regression coefficient is zero, we know the corresponding independent variable has no impact on the dependent variable.

T-test is used to estimate if the overall partial regression coefficient is zero. The hypothesis of the test is

$$H_0: \quad \beta_i = 0$$
$$H_1: \quad \beta_i \neq 0$$
$$\alpha = 0.05.$$

The test statistic is

$$t_{bi} = \frac{b_i}{S_{bi}} \tag{12.5}$$

where S_{bi} is the standard error of i partial regression coefficient. b_i is the partial regression coefficient.

12.3.4 Variable Selection

Not all the supposed independent variables have statistically significant impact on the dependent variable. In many research studies, multiple linear regression aims to build the best predictive regression model. Regression model generally requires bringing variables as much as possible and asks all the impacts of independent variables on the dependent variable are statistically significant. Therefore, we have to select the independent variables and remove the non-significant variables during the multiple linear regression.

The most common methods to select the independent variables are forward selection, backward selection, and stepwise selection. Forward selection is starting with no variables in the model, trying out the variables one by one and including them if they are statistically significant. Backward selection is starting with all candidate variables and testing them one by one for statistical significance, deleting any that are not significant. Stepwise selection is a method that allows moves in either direction, dropping or adding variables at the various steps. The process is one of alternation between choosing the least significant variable to drop and then re-considering all dropped variables (except the most recently dropped) for re-introduction into the model. This means that two separate significance levels must be chosen for deletion from the model and for adding to the model. The second significance must be more stringent than the first.

12.3.5 Collinearity Diagnostics

Except the prerequisite such as linearity, independency, normal distribution, and equal variance, we still need to consider the relation between the independent variables. Multicollinearity exists when the random independent variables are highly related, and it can bring many problems to the regression estimation and inference. For instance, the estimates of the regression coefficients can be instable, which express as a large standard error. In that case, some important but not statistically significant variable cannot be included in the equation; in the serious situations, the sample regression coefficient cannot by explained practically.

The simplest method to deal with multicollinearity is to remove the variables: we remove the variables that have largest standard error, most missing data, and the least important variables among the one that have strong correlation. In addition, we can use the principal component regression method (refer other materials).

12.3.6 Interaction

We already mentioned the concept of interaction in ANOVA of factorial design information. In multiple linear regression, we always consider if the independent variables interact with each other. If the linear relationship between an independent variable and the dependent variable can change with another independent variable, we call the relationship between the two independent variables interaction, which can also be named effect modification.

12.4 Application

Example

A researcher collected the medical records of 77 patients with type 2 diabetes from a hospital between January 2008 and December 2008, and the average age was 62 years old. 40 cases were male and 37 cases were female. Their hepatic and renal function was normal. We selected eight following variables from the medical records: Glycosylated hemoglobin (HbA1c) X_1, Fasting blood-glucose (FBG) X_2. Total cholesterol(TC)X_3, Triglyceride (TG)X_4, High-density lipoprotein cholesterol (HDL-C) X_5, Low-density lipoprotein cholesterol (LDL-C) X_6, Atherosclerosis (AS) X_7, Amyloid-β 40 (Aβ40) Y.

Aβ40 causes the damage of neurons and vascular endothelium as an important risk factor for Alzheimer's disease. Aβ40 is a continuous numerical variable and is followed normal distribution. We can perform multiple linear regression analysis between Y and seven independent variables X_1–X_7 to explore which factors impact on the level of Aβ40 for patients with type 2 diabetes.

12.4.1 Build a SPSS Data File

In the first, we quantify the qualitative variables, like AS X_7: Yes = 1, No = 0.

The process of inputting the data into SPSS is File → Open → Data → select the data location or copy the text data file into SPSS. Then, we can determine the data type and the number of decimal places.

12.4.2 Multiple Linear Regression by SPSS

The main process to show the multiple linear correlations between Y and X_1–X_7 by SPSS 20.0 is

Analyze → Regression → Linear → Y → select to Dependent → X_1, ..., X_p select to Independent(s) → Method → Stepwise → Options → OK.

Step by step process:

1. Analyze → Regression → Linear, enter linear regression model, as shown in Fig. 12.1:
2. In linear regression window, we select the Aβ40 value when discharge Y as dependent, seven independent variables X_1–X_7 as Independent, and chooses Stepwise in Methods. In SPSS20.0, it provides 5 methods to select variables: enter, stepwise, remove, backward, and forward.

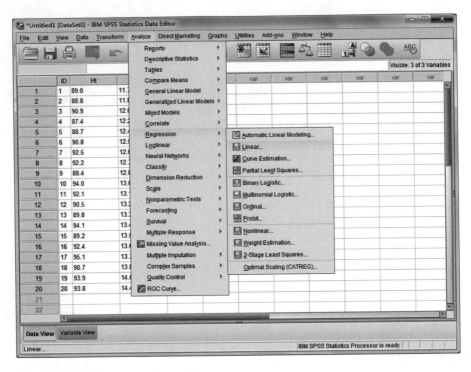

Fig. 12.1 Enter linear regression model

3. Click on statistics. Select estimates, model fit, R squared change, and Durbin–Watson.
4. Click on plots. Select SRESID as y-axis, DEPENDNT as the x-axis, and select Histogram and Normal probability plot.
5. Click on options. Select use probability of F, and input 0.05 in entry and 0.10 in removal (as system default value). Click on continue, and then click on OK.

12.4.3 Main Output Results

Figure 12.2 model summary shows the R square in the two models. We know from the figure that $R = 0.738$ in model 2, $R^2 = 0.545$, adjusted $R^2 = 0.533$, and standard error of the estimate = 169.213.

Figure 12.3 shows the testing results in the two models, and we can look for the F-stat in the last model. $F = 44.361$, $P < 0.001$, when $\alpha = 0.05$. So we can consider there is linear relationship between Y and X_7, X_6.

We can finally obtain the multivariate linear regression equation from the model two shown in Fig. 12.4:

$$\hat{Y} = 6.488 + 305.406X_7 + 108.373X_6$$

Model Summary

Model	R	R Square	Adjusted R Square	Std. Error of the Estimate	Change Statistics				
					R Square Change	F Change	df1	df2	Sig. F Change
1	.693ᵃ	.480	.473	179.760	.480	69.187	1	75	.000
2	.738ᵇ	.545	.533	169.213	.065	10.641	1	74	.002

Fig. 12.2 Model summary show R^2

ANOVAᵃ

Model		Sum of Squares	df	Mean Square	F	Sig.
1	Regression	2235676.600	1	2235676.600	69.187	.000ᵇ
	Residual	2423511.107	75	32313.481		
	Total	4659187.707	76			
2	Regression	2540353.829	2	1270176.914	44.361	.000ᶜ
	Residual	2118833.878	74	28632.890		
	Total	4659187.707	76			

a. Dependent Variable: y

b. Predictors: (Constant), x7

c. Predictors: (Constant), x7, x6

Fig. 12.3 Model Summary show significant testing

Coefficientsᵃ

Model		Unstandardized Coefficients		Standardized Coefficients	t	Sig.
		B	Std. Error	Beta		
1	(Constant)	274.769	29.161		9.423	.000
	x7	340.821	40.974	.693	8.318	.000
2	(Constant)	6.488	86.704		.075	.941
	x7	305.406	40.069	.621	7.622	.000
	x6	108.373	33.223	.266	3.262	.002

a. Dependent Variable: y

Fig. 12.4 Coefficient show the regression coefficient and the hypothesis testing

12.4.4 Conclusion

The level of Aβ40 for patients with type 2 diabetes can be mainly determined by Atherosclerosis and LDL-C. Type 2 diabetes patients with atherosclerosis can be expected a higher level of Aβ40 than those without atherosclerosis. Type 2 diabetes patients with high level of LDL-C can be expected a high level of Aβ40.

Chapter Summary
1. Multiple linear regression analysis is the extension of simple linear regression analysis, with only one response variable, but more than one independent variable. Model assumption and the least squares principle are the same with the simple linear regression analysis.
2. A partial regression coefficient in the model indicates the average amount of change as the certain independent variable changes for one unit when other independent variables were fixed. That is, the partial regression coefficient is the regression effect of certain variable after adjusting for the effects from other independent variables.
3. The partial regression coefficient could be influenced by dimensions, therefore, cannot be used to compare independent factors' impacts for dependent variable. Standardized partial regression coefficient of eliminate the influence for different units; their absolute value could be used to compare their effects on the response variable.
4. Variable selection was used to retain important variables that make more contribution to the regression, to establish a concise model but with higher estimation accuracy.

Chapter 13
Logistic Regression

Wenli Lu and Yuan Wang

Objectives
Binary responses are common in clinical medicine. In this chapter, we will study a model for binary or binomial response. This model focuses on the popular logit model, which is also called Logistic Regression. Significance testing and model interpretation with Odds Ratios are introduced. SPSS software is employed to comply with a Logistic Regression model.

Key Concepts
Logistic Regression; Binary response; Odds Ratio; Logit Transformation

13.1 Introduction

Regression models have been widely used in data analysis concerned with the relationship between one response (dependent) variable and one or more explanatory (independent) variables. The outcome variable is usually binary, such as dead or alive for survival state, and present or absent for disease state. Logistic Regression model has been regarded as a standard analytic approach in such a situation. In this chapter, we will introduce the principles and applications of the Logistic Regression model.

W. Lu (✉) · Y. Wang
School of Public Health, Tianjin Medical University, Tianjin, China
e-mail: luwenli@tmu.edu.cn

© Zhengzhou University Press 2024
X. Guo, F. Xue (eds.), *Textbook of Medical Statistics*,
https://doi.org/10.1007/978-981-99-7390-3_13

13.2   Logistic Regression

13.2.1   From Linear Regression to Logistic Regression

Principles of linear regression will also guide Logistic Regression. For the regression problem, linear regression can be illustrated as:

$$E(Y|x) = \beta_0 + \beta_1 x \qquad (13.1)$$

E($Y|x$) is the conditional mean of Y, given the value x. With the binary outcome, E($Y|x$) must be in the interval 0–1 ($0 \leq E(Y|x) \leq 1$). To simplify notation, we use $\pi(x) = E(Y|x)$ to represent the mean of Y given x when the binary outcome is used. The equation of the Logistic Regression model is as follows:

$$\pi(x) = \frac{e^{\beta_0 + \beta_1 x}}{1 + e^{\beta_0 + \beta_1 x}}. \qquad (13.2)$$

In linear regression, the outcome can be expressed as $y = E(Y|x) + \varepsilon$. ε is called error which means the deviation of y from E($Y|x$) and it follows a normal distribution. For a binary outcome, $y = \pi(x) + \varepsilon$, where ε may assume one of two results:
   If $y = 1$, $\varepsilon = 1 - \pi(x)$;
   If $y = 0$, $\varepsilon = -\pi(x)$.
   Therefore, ε follows a distribution with a mean of zero and a variance of $\pi(x)[1 - \pi(x)]$, which is a binomial distribution.
   Thus, when we see the binary outcome in a regression model:

1. Conditional mean E($Y|x$) must be in the interval 0–1;
2. The binomial distribution is the basis of Logistic Regression;
3. Principles in linear regression will also guide Logistic Regression.

13.2.2   Logit Transformation

A transformation of $\pi(x)$, which plays a crucial role in logistic regression, is called logit transformation and is defined as:

$$g(x) = In\left[\frac{\pi(x)}{1 - \pi(x)}\right] = \beta_0 + \beta_1 x. \qquad (13.3)$$

The logit $g(x)$ has similar properties with a linear regression model, which is continuous and has a range of $-\infty \sim +\infty$, depending on the value of x.

13.2.3 Odds and Logit Transformation

In formula (13.3), $\dfrac{\pi(x)}{(1-\pi(x))}$ is called the odds of the event, which is represented by the probability of the event happening, $\pi(x)$, divided by the probability of the event not happening $1 - \pi(x)$. The range of $\pi(x)$ and $1 - \pi(x)$ is between 0 and 1. With the logit link function $g(x)$, the log odds has a linear relationship with independent variables.

13.3 Logistic Regression Model

13.3.1 Estimation and Interpretation of Regression Coefficients

The coefficient β for an independent variable represents the magnitude by which the dependent variable will change if the independent variable changes by one unit. In the Logistic Regression model, we assume that the independent variable x is coded 1 or 0. The difference, which is in logit form, between an individual with $x = 1$ and another individual with $x = 0$ is expressed as:

$$g(1)-g(0)=[\beta_0+\beta_1]-[\beta_0]=\beta_1.$$

To get the meaning of β, the first thing is to introduce the term Odds Ratio. The odds of $x = 1$ is $\pi(1)/[1 - \pi(1)]$ and the odds of $x = 0$ is $\pi(0)/[1 - \pi(0)]$. Therefore, the Odds Ratio, which is commonly represented as OR, is expressed as the ratio of the odds of $x = 1$ to the odds of $x = 0$, and can be written as follows:

$$OR = \frac{\pi(1)/[1-\pi(1)]}{\pi(0)/[1-\pi(0)]}. \tag{13.4}$$

Substituting the expression of a Logistic Regression model with Eq. (13.3), we get the results in Table 13.1.

Table 13.1 The relationship between Y and x in the logistic model

Dependent variable (Y)	Independent variable (x)	
	$x = 1$	$x = 0$
$y = 1$	$\pi(1) = \dfrac{e^{\beta_0+\beta_1}}{1+e^{\beta_0+\beta_1}}$	$\pi(0) = \dfrac{e^{\beta_0}}{1+e^{\beta_0}}$
$y = 0$	$1-\pi(1) = \dfrac{1}{1+e^{\beta_0+\beta_1}}$	$1-\pi(0) = \dfrac{1}{1+e^{\beta_0}}$

$$OR = \frac{\left(\dfrac{e^{\beta_0+\beta_1}}{1+e^{\beta_0+\beta_1}}\right)\bigg/\left(\dfrac{1}{1+e^{\beta_0+\beta_1}}\right)}{\left(\dfrac{e^{\beta_0}}{1+e^{\beta_0}}\right)\bigg/\left(\dfrac{1}{1+e^{\beta_0}}\right)}$$

$$= \frac{e^{\beta_0+\beta_1}}{e^{\beta_0}}$$

$$= e^{(\beta_0+\beta_1)-\beta_0}$$

$$= e^{\beta_1}$$

The Odds Ratio (OR) is a measure of the relationship between factors and outcome and is widely used in epidemiology. It means how much more likely it is for the outcome event to happen among individuals with $x = 1$ than among individuals with $x = 0$. When $\beta = 0$ and OR = 1, indicating the independent variable x does not affect the dependent variable Y. When $\beta > 0$ and OR > 1, indicating that x has a positive relationship with Y. When $\beta < 0$ and OR < 1, indicating x has a negative relationship with Y.

13.3.2 Hypothesis Testing of Equations

Suppose there is a sample of m records (x_i, Y_i), $i = 1,2,\ldots, m$, x_i is the independent variable and Y_i represents the binary outcome for the ith record (in Logistic Regression, dependent variable can be binary, ordinal, or nominal when the level is greater than 2, but we only discuss the binary situation in this chapter). Y_i is coded as 0 or 1, representing the absence or presence of the outcome. Then, we will comply with the logistic model (13.2) with a dataset and estimate the unknown parameters of β_0 and β_1.

Maximum likelihood method is a general procedure to estimate the parameters in the regression model. In Logistic Regression, maximum likelihood estimation finds the best linear combination of independent variables to maximize the likelihood of obtaining the observed outcome. The first step is to build a likelihood function, which represents the probability of the sample data as a function of unknown parameters. Estimators of the parameters through maximum likelihood method will end up with values that maximize the function. The final estimators are the ones that make $E(Y|x)$ closest to the observed y. The following shows how to use the maximum likelihood method in the Logistic Regression model.

When Y is coded as 0 or 1, $\pi(x)$ in the Eq. (13.2) provides the conditional probability of $Y = 1$ given x, expressed as $P(Y = 1|x)$. $1 - \pi(x)$ represents the conditional probability of $Y = 0$ given x, expressed as $P(Y = 0|x)$. For any record (x_i, Y_i), its contribution to the likelihood function can be expressed as:

if $y_i = 1$, contribution to the likelihood function is $\pi(x_i)$;

if $y_i = 0$, contribution to the likelihood function is $1-\pi(x_i)$.
For convenience, the likelihood function is written as:

$$\pi\left(x_i\right)^{y_i}\left[1-\pi\left(x_i\right)\right]^{1-y_i}. \tag{13.5}$$

Because the records are independent, the likelihood function is expressed as the product of the terms in the following equation:

$$l\left(\beta\right)=\prod_{i=1}^{m}\pi\left(x_i\right)^{y_i}\left[1-\pi\left(x_i\right)\right]^{1-y_i}. \tag{13.6}$$

The log-likelihood function is as follows:

$$L\left(\beta\right)=\ln\left[l\left(\beta\right)\right]=\sum_{m}^{i=1}\left\{y_i\ln\left[\pi\left(x_i\right)\right]+\left(1-y_i\right)\ln\left[1-\pi\left(x_i\right)\right]\right\}. \tag{13.7}$$

To get the estimation of β, $L(\beta)$ should be maximized. Statistical software like SPSS has a special iterative procedure for the estimation of β, which is also called the maximum likelihood estimate $\hat{\beta}$.

13.3.3 Hypothesis Testing of Coefficients

After estimating the coefficients of the fitted model, the next step is to evaluate the significance of the factors. It is a statistical hypothesis to determine whether the independent variable x in the model can explain part of the variation of the dependent variable Y.

In Logistic Regression, likelihood test is usually taken to test the statistical significance of coefficients, by comparing the values of likelihood functions between two models. Model A, which is without the independent variable, has likelihood function value $\ln L_A$. Model B, which is with the independent variable, has likelihood function value $\ln L_B$. The statistic of likelihood function test is expressed as:

$$G=-2\left(\ln L_B-\ln L_A\right) \tag{13.8}$$

G follows a χ^2 distribution. If $G>\chi^2_{\alpha,m}$, this independent x is statistically significant.

$Wald\chi^2$ test is another method to test the significance of coefficient in the logistic model, with a formula as:

$$Wald\,\chi^2=\left(\frac{\beta}{S_\beta}\right)^2 \tag{13.9}$$

β is the partial regression coefficient, S_β is the standard error for β. When a hypothesis is true, $Wald\chi^2$ follows a χ^2 distribution with degree of freedom equal to 1.

13.3.4   Confidence Interval Estimation of Coefficient

The sample distribution of estimated parameter follows a normal distribution. According to the principle of normal distribution, the confidence interval of β at $(1-\alpha)$ level is $\beta \pm Z_{\alpha/2}S_\beta$. In Logistic Regression, the value of OR is e^β, with $(1-\alpha)$ confidence interval $e^{(\beta \pm Z_{\alpha/2}S_\beta)}$.

13.3.5   Model Selection

When there are many independent variables in the regression model, it is necessary to select variables with statistically significant contribution and delete those with little contribution to the variation of the dependent variable. In Logistic Regression, forward selection and backward selection are common methods for model selection.

13.4   Applications

13.4.1   Build a SPSS Data File

Example 13.1 To investigate the risk factors for diabetes, a survey was conducted among 60 residences. The code of risk factors is given in Table 13.2.

13.4.2   Logistic Regression Using SPSS

In this section, we will examine the relationship between Diabetes (Y) and 7 independent variables x_1–x_7. In SPSS 20.0 (IBM SPSS Statistics 20.0), the procedure of analysis is as follows:

Table 13.2 The code of risk factors

Risk factors	Variable	Code
Age (years)	x_1	Continuous
Family history of diabetes	x_2	No = 0, Yes = 1
Smoke	x_3	No = 0, Yes = 1
Drink	x_4	No = 0, Yes = 1
Body mass index (BMI) category	x_5	Normal = 1, overweight = 2, obesity = 3
Sport exercise	x_6	No = 0, Yes = 1
Character	x_7	A = 0, B = 1
Diabetes	Y	No = 0, Yes = 1

1. Open dataset 13.1.sav.
2. Analyze → Regression → Binary Logistic and Open Logistic Regression box.
3. In the Logistic Regression box, select Y into Dependent box and x_1-x_7 into Covariates box. In Method option, SPSS provides 7 methods for the selection of independent variables:

    (1) Enter (select all independent variables); (2) Forward: Conditional (Forward selection: select independent variables according to conditional parameter likelihood ratio test); (3) Forward: LR (Forward selection: select independent variables according to partial maximum likelihood ratio test); (4) Forward: Wald (Forward selection: select independent variables according to Wald statistic); (5) Backward: Conditional (Backward selection: select independent variables according to conditional parameter likelihood ratio test); (6) Backward: LR (Backward selection: select independent variables according to partial maximum likelihood ratio test); (7) Backward: Wald (Backward selection: select independent variables according to Wald statistic). For this example, we choose Enter (Fig. 13.1).

4. If the independent variable is categorical variable, like BMI category (normal, overweight, obesity), which has no linear relationship with the dependent variable, it is necessary to transform the categorical variable of K level into K-1 dummy variables. In the Logistic Regression box, click Categorical and it will display Logistic Regression: Define Categorical Variables box. Put X5 (BMI) into Categorical Covariates box, select First in Change Contrast, then click change button. Click continue and return to Logistic Regression box Fig. 13.1 Logistic Regression model

5. In the Logistic Regression box, click Options, and it will display Logistic Regression: Options box. Select CI for EXP(B): 95% box and put 0.05 into Entry box, 0.10 into Remove box (they are the default values in SPSS 22, which can be modified in the application). Click Continue and return to Logistic Regression box. Click OK to start the analysis.

Variables in the Equation

		B	S.E.	Wald	df	Sig.	Exp(B)	95% C.I.for EXP(B)	
								Lower	Upper
Step 1[a]	X1	.058	.032	3.317	1	.069	1.060	.996	1.128
	X2	2.114	.878	5.805	1	.016	8.285	1.483	46.274
	X3	.208	1.037	.040	1	.841	1.232	.161	9.404
	X4	−.682	1.122	.370	1	.543	.506	.056	4.558
	X5			6.224	2	.045			
	X5(1)	.839	.969	.749	1	.387	2.313	.346	15.454
	X5(2)	2.956	1.188	6.192	1	.013	19.216	1.873	197.117
	X6	−.190	.893	.045	1	.831	.827	.144	4.761
	X7	.414	.857	.234	1	.629	1.513	.282	8.115
	Constant	−5.695	1.786	10.165	1	.001	.003		

a. Variable(s) entered on step 1: X1, X2, X3, X4, X5, X6, X7.

Fig. 13.1 Results of variables in the equation

13.4.3 Main Output Results

In this example, we use Enter method and put all variables into the model. Finally, x_2 (family history of diabetes) and x_5 (BMI) are significantly associated with Y (diabetes) with $P < 0.05$.

In the previous section, we mentioned that SPSS 20.0 has seven methods to select independent variables. Now, we will try Forward: Conditional methods. The procedure is as follows:

Analyze → Regression → Binary Logistic → Y enter Dependent → $X_1...X_7$ enter Covariates → Method → Forward: Conditional → Categorical, select x_5 → Options, select CI for exp(B) 95% → Continue → OK.

The result of Forward: Conditional is similar to that of Enter. Here shows some important parts.

Figure 13.2 shows that in forward: conditional method, after two steps of selection, x_2 (family history of diabetes) and X_5 (BMI) enter the final model ($P < 0.05$), which is consistent with the result of enter method.

13.4.4 Conclusion

In multiple Logistic Regression, a family history of diabetes (OR = 6.47, $P = 0.016$) and obesity (OR = 23.681, $P = 0.004$) is significantly associated with the presence of diabetes, that is, the odds of a family history of diabetes among cases are 6.47 times greater than that of the odds of a family history of diabetes among the controls. For obesity, the odds of obesity among cases are 23,681 times greater than the odds of obesity among the controls. They may be risk factors for diabetes, indicating that subjects with a family history of diabetes and obesity should pay attention to diabetes prevention.

Variables in the Equation

		B	S.E.	Wald	df	Sig.	Exp(B)	95% C.I.for EXP(B)	
								Lower	Upper
Step 1[a]	X5			10.962	2	.004			
	X5(1)	1.170	.797	2.158	1	.142	3.222	.676	15.352
	X5(2)	3.367	1.017	10.961	1	.001	29.000	3.950	212.888
	Constant	−2.269	.606	13.993	1	.000	.103		
Step 2[b]	X2	1.867	.772	5.844	1	.016	6.471	1.424	29.407
	X5			8.415	2	.015			
	X5(1)	1.327	.857	2.394	1	.122	3.768	.702	20.230
	X5(2)	3.165	1.096	8.330	1	.004	23.681	2.761	203.114
	Constant	−3.035	.775	15.334	1	.000	.048		

a. Variable(s) entered on step 1: X5.

b. Variable(s) entered on step 2: X2.

Fig. 13.2 Results of variables in the equation

Chapter Summary
1. Principles in linear regression will also guide Logistic Regression. The difference is that the outcome dependent variable is continuous in linear regression but is binary in Logistic Regression.
2. Logit Transformation builds a linear relationship between the Odds Ratio and independent variables. The Odds Ratio is a practical measure to interpret the relationship between independent variables and dependent variable.
3. Likelihood ratio test is usually used to test the overall significance of the fitted Logistic Regression model. $Wald\chi^2$ test is applied to test the significance of independent variables in the model.

Chapter 14
Survival Analysis

Hongmei Yu and Yan Guo

Objectives

In logistic regression, we are interested in how risk factors are associated with the presence or absence of an event. Sometimes, however, we are interested in how a risk factor or treatment affects the time to the event. The problem of analyzing time to event data arises in a number of applied fields, such as medicine, public health, and epidemiology. Survival analysis is a collection of statistical methods that are used to describe, explain, or predict the occurrence and timing of events. This chapter focuses on basic concepts of survival analysis, survival rate estimation, comparison of survival curves, and SPSS software procedures.

Key Concepts

Survival analysis; Survival time; Censoring; Survival function; Survival curve; Kaplan–Meier method; Log-rank test

H. Yu (✉)
School of Public Health, Shanxi Medical University, Taiyuan, China

Y. Guo
School of Public Health, Sun Yat-sen University, Guangzhou, China

© Zhengzhou University Press 2024
X. Guo, F. Xue (eds.), *Textbook of Medical Statistics*,
https://doi.org/10.1007/978-981-99-7390-3_14

14.1 Basic Concepts

14.1.1 Survival Time

Survival time or time to event refers to the duration from a clear and well-defined starting point to the occurrence of the outcome of interest. The starting point may be the date of first diagnosis, admission to hospital, or starting treatment in a randomized controlled trial. The outcome of interest can be death, recurrence of the tumor, the first occurrence of a particular complication, etc., which can be a single event or composite events. Examples of survival time are the time from surgical excision to death in patients with bladder cancer; the time from drug chemotherapy to complete remission or partial remission in patients with acute leukemia; the time from the disappearance of positive signs to the first relapse in women with hyperplasia of mammary glands through drug treatment. Overall survival (OS) and progression-free survival (PFS), which are common measures of survival time in clinical trials, are widely used in composite events. OS generally refers to the period from the date of group randomization to death for any reason; PFS generally refers to the time from group randomization to the pre-identified disease progression, such as distant metastasis of a tumor, secondary primary tumor, or death. Survival time is also known as failure time and can be measured in years, weeks, days, hours, etc.

During the follow-ups, researchers might observe a given end-point event in some subjects, and these exact survival time data are called complete data of survival time. Observations are called censoring when the information about their survival time is incomplete, of which the most common form is right censoring. Three common situations where an individual's survival time is right-censored are: an individual does not experience the event before the study ends, an individual is lost to follow-up during the study period, or an individual withdraws from the study. Censored survival time is measured from the starting point to the point of censoring. Right censoring means the actual survival time is longer than the censored time, often marked with "+" on the upper right of the case. Although censored observations are incomplete, their survival time up to the point of censorship can provide useful information. Censoring that is random and non-informative is usually required to avoid bias in survival analysis.

Survival data have three common features that are difficult to handle with conventional statistical methods and make survival analysis distinct from other types of analysis: (1) focusing on time to the event; (2) containing censored observations; and (3) skewed survival time data not suitable for the application of the usual methods based on normal data.

14.1.2 Probability of Death and Survival

During a specific time interval, the probability of death is the conditional probability that someone who survives exactly t will die before reaching time $(t+1)$ (e.g., annual probability of death is the probability that the surviving population at the beginning of the year will die by the end of the year)

$$q = \frac{\text{number of living during the time interval}}{\text{number alive at the beginning of time}}. \tag{14.1}$$

The probability of survival is the conditional probability that someone who survives exact t will survive to time $(t+1)$ (e.g., annual probability of survival is the probability that the surviving population at the beginning of the year will survive this year)

$$p = \frac{\text{number of living during the time interval}}{\text{number alive at the beginning of time}}. \tag{14.2}$$

If the observation period is the same, then $p = 1 - q$.

14.1.3   Survival Function and Hazard Function

Survival function refers to the probability that an individual will survive beyond a specific point in time t, which is denoted by $S(t)$, $0 \le S(t) \le 1$. The survival function summarizes information of survival data by giving survival probabilities to different time points. For complete data, the survival function can be directly estimated as:

$$S(t) = P(T > t) = \frac{\text{number of living at time } t}{\text{number alive at the beginning of time}}. \tag{14.3}$$

While for censored data, the survival function is the product of conditional probabilities of survival:

$$S(t_k) = P(T > t_k) = p_1 \cdot p_2 \cdots p_k = S(t_{k-1}) \cdot p_k \tag{14.4}$$

where $p_i(i=1, 2, \ldots, k)$ is the conditional probability of survival for each time interval, so the survival function is also called cumulative survival rate.

If the end-point event is death, the hazard function describes the risk of death in an interval after time t, conditional on the subject having survived to time t, denoted by $h(t)$.

$$h(t) = \lim_{\Delta t \to 0} \frac{P(t \le T < t + \Delta t | T \ge t)}{\Delta t} \tag{14.5}$$

The hazard function can be thought of as the instantaneous risk that an event will take place at time t given that the subject has survived to time t, which is also known as the instantaneous failure rate, the force of mortality, conditional mortality rate, and age-specific failure rate. Note that $h(t)$ is rate rather than probability, and the range is 0 to $+\infty$. In contrast to the survival function, the hazard function summarizes survival data by focusing on the failures. The survival analysis model is usually given in the form of $h(t)$, see Chap. 15 for details.

14.1.4   Survival Curve, Hazard Curve, and Median Survival Time

The survival curve is the plot of survival function $S(t)$ (vertical axis) against t (horizontal axis). The survival curve is a descending curve. We should pay attention to the height of the curve and the descending slope, with a higher and flatter curve indicating better survival. The hazard curve is the plot of hazard function $h(t)$ (vertical axis) against t (horizontal axis).

The median survival time indicates the time at which exactly 50% of individuals survive (i.e., the time at which the survival curve reaches 50%). The longer the median survival time, the better the prognosis of the disease, and vice versa. Estimating median survival time often uses graphical or linear interpolation method.

14.2   Estimation of Survival Function

Cumulative survival probabilities can be estimated by using either the Kaplan–Meier method or the lifetable method. Both of them follow the basic principle of cohort life table and calculate the survival rate based on the product of the conditional probability of survival. The former applies to either large or small sample data containing individual survival times; the latter applies to large sample data grouped by time intervals.

14.2.1   Kaplan–Meier Estimates

The Kaplan–Meier estimator of the survival function, also called the product limit estimator, is the default estimator used by most software packages. "Product": the cumulative survival rate is a product of the conditional probability of survival; "Limit": the Kaplan–Meier estimates are limited to the time interval in which the observations fall.

Example 14.1 Survival times (in weeks) of 20 patients with a brain tumor were collected, and survival function was needed to estimate.

Treatment Group A	5	7+	13	13	23	30	30+	38	42	42	45+
Treatment Group B	1	3	3	7	10	15	15	23	30		

Survival data for treatment group A are ungrouped small sample data containing censoring, and the survival function estimates are presented in Table 14.1.

1. Rank the survival time (t_i) in ascending order. If the complete survival time is the same as the censored time, the censored time should be listed after the complete time, as given in column (2) in Table 14.1.

Table 14.1 The survival function estimates for treatment group A

ID	Time (weeks)	Number of deaths	Number of censored	Number at risk	Probability of death	Probability of survival	Cumulative survival rate	Standard error of survival rate
i	t_i	d_i	c_i	n_i	$\hat{q}_i$	$\hat{p}_i$	$\hat{S}(t_i)$	$SE\left[\hat{S}(t_i)\right]$
(1)	(2)	(3)	(4)	(5)	(6)	(7)	(8)	(9)
1	5	1	0	11	1/11 = 0.0909	0.9091	0.9091	0.0867
2	7	0	1	10	0/11 = 0.0000	1.0000	0.9091 × 1.0000 = 0.9091	0.0867
3	13	2	0	9	2/9 = 0.2222	0.7778	0.9091 × 0.7778 = 0.7071	0.1429
4	23	1	0	7	1/7 = 0.1429	0.8571	0.7071 × 0.8571 = 0.6061	0.1541
5	30	1	0	6	1/6 = 0.1667	0.8333	0.6061 × 0.8333 = 0.5051	0.1581
6	30	0	1	5	0/5 = 0.0000	1.0000	0.5051 × 1.0000 = 0.5051	0.1581
7	38	1	0	4	1/4 = 0.2500	0.7500	0.5051 × 0.7500 = 0.3788	0.1613
8	42	2	0	3	2/3 = 0.6667	0.3333	0.3788 × 0.3333 = 0.1263	0.1163
9	45	0	1	1	0/1 = 0.0000	1.0000	0.1263 × 1.0000 = 0.1263	0.1163

2. List the number of deaths d_i and the number of censored c_i in time interval $[t_i, t_{i+1})$, as given in columns (3) and (4) in Table 14.1.

3. Calculate the number at risk n_i (i.e., number alive at the beginning of t_i). The number of deaths and censored before t_i should be subtracted (i.e., $n_i = n_{i-1} - d_{i-1} - c_{i-1}$). See column (5) in Table 14.1.

4. Calculate the conditional probability of death $\hat{q}_i$ and the conditional probability of survival $\hat{p}_i$ at each time interval, see columns (6) and (7) in Table 14.1.

5. Calculate the cumulative survival rate $\hat{S}(t_i)$ according to formula (14.4), see Table 14.1 column (8). Results showed a 90.91% probability of 5-week survival after treatment A for patients with brain tumor and the survival rate of 13 weeks was 70.71% and so on. Survival rate does not change at censored time as censored time only provides information to the number at risk.

The Kaplan–Meier survival curve is a stepped line since the cumulative survival rate drops at the precise time that death occurs and remains constant between successive death times. The survival curves for patients with brain tumor in group A and group B (calculation table omitted) are shown in Fig. 14.1a, and the hazard curves are shown in Fig. 14.1b. The median survival times were 38 (weeks) and 10 (weeks), respectively.

14.2.2 Life Table Estimation

In some cohort studies, we do not know the exact time of death or censoring of individuals (e.g., the death or censoring of certain individuals at follow-up occurs between two visits at a tumor registry or from other large surveillance systems). The life table method is a classical way to analyze grouped survival data.

Example 14.2 A total of 374 patients with malignant tumor were followed and grouped at each time interval of 1 year. The information needed to estimate the cumulative survival rate is given in columns (1)–(5) in Table 14.2.

1. Calculate the effective number at risk n_i. It is assumed that the time to loss or withdrawal is approximately uniformly distributed in the interval. Therefore, people lost or withdrawn in the interval are exposed to the risk of death for one-half of the interval, i.e., $n_i = n_i' - c_i / 2$. See column (6) in Table 14.2.
2. Calculate the probability of death $\hat{q}_i$ and the probability of survival $\hat{p}_i$ of each time interval.

$$\hat{q}_i = \frac{d_i}{n_i' - c_i / 2} = \frac{d_i}{n_i} \quad \hat{p}_i = 1 - \hat{q}_i \tag{14.6}$$

See columns (7) and (8) in Table 14.2.
3. Calculate the cumulative survival rate according to formula (14.4), see Table 14.2 column (9). Results showed that the one-year survival rate of patients with the malignant tumor was 75.94%, the 2-year survival rate was 55.62%, and so on.

Survival curve and hazard curve are shown in Fig. 14.2a, b, respectively. This indicates that malignant tumor poses a greater threat to the patients' survival within 5 years of diagnosis. The median survival time was 2.4 (years).

14.2.3 Interval Estimation of Survival Rate

The survival rate $\hat{S}(t_i)$ calculated from the sample data is a point estimate based on which the overall survival rate can be estimated. Standard error approximation formula of Greenwood is

Table 14.2 Life table estimation of survival rate

ID	Years after diagnosis	Number of deaths in the year	Number of censored during the year	Number at risk	Effective number at risk	Probability of death	Probability of survival	Cumulative survival rate	Standard error of survival rate
i	$t_i\sim$	d_i	c_i	n_i'	n_i	$\hat{q}_i$	$\hat{p}_i$	$\hat{S}(t_i)$	$SE\left[\hat{S}(t_i)\right]$
(1)	(2)	(3)	(4)	(5)	(6)	(7)	(8)	(9)	(10)
1	0~	90	0	374	374.0	$90/374.0 = 0.2406$	0.7594	0.7594	0.0221
2	1~	76	0	284	284.0	$76/284.0 = 0.2676$	0.7324	$0.7594 \times 0.7324 = 0.5562$	0.0257
3	2~	51	0	208	208.0	$51/208.0 = 0.2452$	0.7548	$0.5562 \times 0.7548 = 0.4198$	0.0255
4	3~	25	12	157	151.0	$25/151.0 = 0.1656$	0.8344	$0.4198 \times 0.8344 = 0.3503$	0.0248
5	4~	20	5	120	117.5	$20/117.5 = 0.1702$	0.8298	$0.3503 \times 0.8298 = 0.2907$	0.0239
6	5~	7	9	95	90.5	$7/90.5 = 0.0773$	0.9227	$0.2907 \times 0.9227 = 0.2682$	0.0235
7	6~	4	9	79	74.5	$4/74.5 = 0.0537$	0.9463	$0.2682 \times 0.9463 = 0.2538$	0.0233
8	7~	1	3	66	64.5	$1/64.5 = 0.0155$	0.9845	$0.2538 \times 0.9845 = 0.2499$	0.0233
9	8~	3	5	62	59.5	$3/59.5 = 0.0504$	0.9496	$0.2499 \times 0.9496 = 0.2373$	0.0232
10	9~10	2	5	54	51.5	$2/51.5 = 0.0388$	0.9612	$0.2373 \times 0.9612 = 0.2281$	0.0232

Note: 47 cases have a survival time of more than 10 years

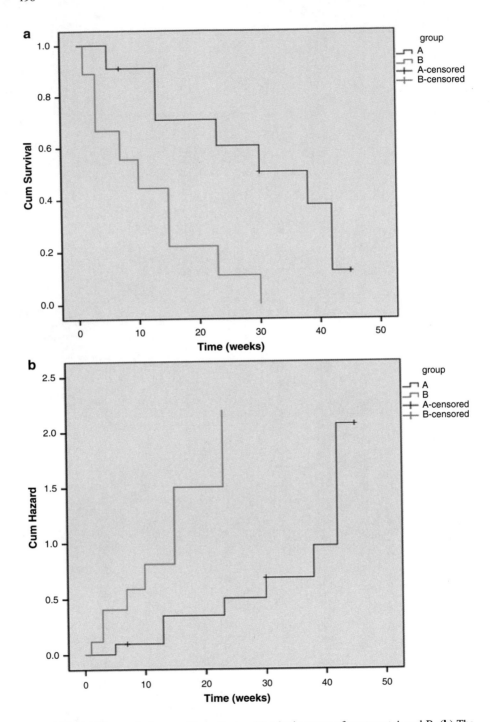

Fig. 14.1 (**a**) The survival curves for patients with a brain tumor of treatment A and B. (**b**) The hazard curves for patients with a brain tumor of treatment A and B

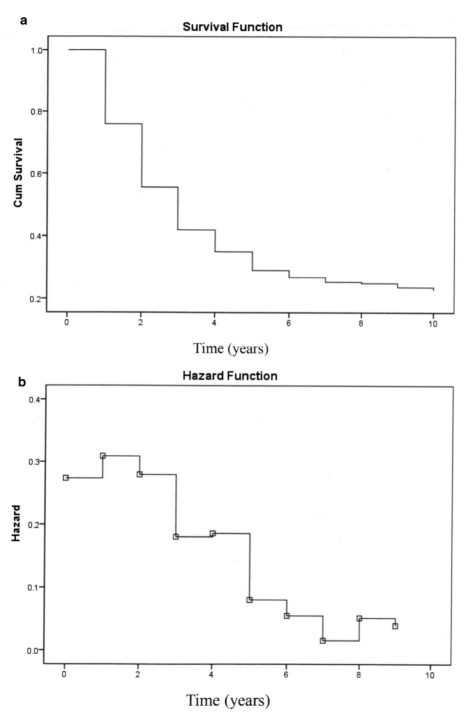

Fig. 14.2 (**a**) Survival curve of patients with malignant tumor. (**b**) Hazard curve of patients with malignant tumor

$$SE\left[\hat{S}(t_i)\right] = \hat{S}(t_i)\sqrt{\sum_{t_j \le t_i} \frac{d_j}{n_j\left(n_j - d_j\right)}}. \tag{14.7}$$

The survival rate is approximately normally distributed for a larger sample and the $(1-\alpha)$confidence interval of the overall survival rate is

$$\hat{S}(t_i) \pm Z_{\alpha/2} \cdot SE\left[\hat{S}(t_i)\right] \tag{14.8}$$

where $Z_{\alpha/2}$ is the critical value of the standard normal distribution corresponding to the two-sided area α, when $\alpha = 0.05$, $Z_{0.05/2} = 1.96$.

Standard error of $\hat{S}(t_4)$ in Table 14.1 is

$$SE\left[\hat{S}(t_4)\right] = 0.6061 \times \sqrt{\frac{1}{11 \times 10} + \frac{2}{9 \times 7} + \frac{1}{7 \times 6}} = 0.1541.$$

The 95% confidence interval of the overall survival rate is $0.6061 \pm 1.96 \times 0.1541$ = $(0.3041, 0.9081)$.

14.3 Comparison of Survival Curves

14.3.1 Log-Rank Test

In many situations, the primary objective of the study is to compare the survival experience of different groups of patients. These groups may be defined according to gender, stage of the tumor at the time of diagnosis, histological type, etc. In clinical trials, groups will be defined by the treatment given. Cumulative survival probabilities are calculated separately for each group, and the two survival curves are plotted on the same graph for comparison (Fig. 14.1a). Statistical tests for the formal comparison of the two survival curves, such as the log-rank test, can then be used to assess the statistical significance of any observed differences.

Example 14.3 Compare the survival curves of patients with brain tumor in treatment group A and B in Example 14.1.

$$H_0 : S_1(t) = S_2(t), \text{for all } t > 0$$

$$H_1 : S_1(t) \ne S_2(t), \text{for some } t > 0$$

$$\alpha = 0.05.$$

The basic idea of the log-rank test: we can calculate the expected number of deaths in each group according to the mortality rate at time point t_i under H_0 and get the total expected deaths T_{gi} in each group. The statistic for the log-rank test is calculated by comparing the observed number of deaths d_{gi} with the expected number of deaths T_{gi} in each group

$$\chi^2 = \frac{\left[\Sigma\left(d_{gi} - T_{gi}\right)\right]^2}{V_g} \quad v = k-1 \tag{14.9}$$

where V_g is the estimate of the variance of the expected number in group g,
$V_g = \Sigma \frac{n_{gi}}{n_i}\left(1 - \frac{n_{gi}}{n_i}\right)\left(\frac{n_i - d_i}{n_i - 1}\right)d_i$. This statistic follows χ^2 distribution with $(k-1)$
degrees of freedom where k is the number of groups.

1. Rank the survival time (t_i) in ascending order, as shown in column (1) in Table 14.3.
2. List the number at risk n_{gi} and the number of deaths d_{gi} at time t_i in each group, see column (2), (3), (6), and (7) in Table 14.3. The total number at risk n_i and deaths d_i are given in columns (10) and (11) in Table 14.3.

3. Calculate the expected number of deaths T_{gi} at time t_i in each group (columns (4) and (8) in Table 14.3). The formula is the same as the formula in Chap. 9

$$T_{gi} = \frac{n_{gi}d_i}{n_i}. \tag{14.10}$$

A single 2×2 table is created for each unique and complete survival time t_i as given in Table 14.4 taking the first time point (1 week) as an example. The

Table 14.3 Log-rank test of comparing survival curves of two treatments

Time(weeks)	Treatment A				Treatment B				Total	
t_i	d_{1i}	n_{1i}	$T_{1i} = n_{1i}d_i/n_i$	V_{1i}	d_{2i}	n_{2i}	$T_{2i} = n_{2i}d_i/n_i$	V_{2i}	d_i	n_i
(1)	(2)	(3)	(4)	(5)	(6)	(7)	(8)	(9)	(10)	(11)
1	0	11	0.5500	0.2475	1	9	0.4500	0.2475	1	20
3	0	11	0.1579	0.4604	2	8	0.8421	0.4604	2	19
5	1	11	0.6471	0.2284	0	6	0.3529	0.2284	1	17
7	0	10	0.6250	0.2344	1	6	0.3750	0.2344	1	16
10	0	9	0.6429	0.2296	1	5	0.3571	0.2296	1	14
13	2	9	1.3846	0.3905	0	4	0.6154	0.3905	2	13
15	0	7	1.2727	0.4165	2	4	0.7273	0.4165	2	11
23	1	7	1.5556	0.3025	1	2	0.4444	0.3025	2	9
30	1	6	1.7143	0.2041	1	1	0.2857	0.2041	2	7
38	1	4	1.0000	0	0	0	0.0000	0	1	4
42	2	3	2.0000	0	0	0	0.0000	0	2	3
Total	8	–	12.5501	2.7139	9	–	4.4499	2.7139	17	–

expected numbers of death for group A and B are $11 \times 1/20 = 0.5500$ and $9 \times 1/20 = 0.4500$, respectively.

4. Calculate the total number of observed and expected deaths in each group. For group A, observed deaths $A_1 = 8$, expected death $T_1 = 12.5501$; for group B, $A_2 = 9$, $T_2 = 4.4499$. $A_1 + A_2 = T_1 + T_2 = 17$, which can be used to double check the result of the calculation.
5. Calculate the estimation of variance V_{gi} shown in column (5) and column (9) in Table 14.3 and $V_1 = V_2 = 2.7139$.
6. Calculate the statistic.

$$\chi^2 = \frac{(8 - 12.5501)^2}{2.7139} = \frac{(9 - 4.4499)^2}{2.7139} = 7.628$$

$v = 1, 0.01 < P < 0.025.$ We reject the H_0 and conclude that the survival curve of the treatment group A is higher than that of the treatment group B.

14.3.2 Practical Notes

1. If the time interval is small enough to cause deaths in each interval $d_k \leq 1$, the test of the H_0 depends only on the order of the occurrence of death rather than the time at which death occurs. Therefore, the log-rank statistic is a rank-based test statistic, hence the name of the log-rank test.
2. Log-rank test is a univariate test. When comparing survival curves in relation to a particular prognostic factor, it is important to ensure that the groups are similar in relation to other prognostic factors.
3. Occasionally, we are interested in comparing g survival curves at a predetermined fixed point at time t_0. For example, one may wish to compare the survival curves at 3 years. Normalized approximation methods can be applied

$$Z = \frac{\hat{S}_1(t) - \hat{S}_2(t)}{\sqrt{SE^2\left[\hat{S}_1(t)\right] + SE^2\left[\hat{S}_2(t)\right]}}. \tag{14.11}$$

Table 14.4 Calculation table of expected deaths (taking the first time as an example)

Group	Dead	Alive	Total (at risk)
Group A	0	11	11
Group B	1	8	9
Total	1	19	20

If one is interested in comparing survival curves at multiple time points, the test level should be corrected by Bonferroni method (i.e., $\alpha' = \alpha/k$), where k is the number of comparisons ensuring that the total type I error does not exceed α.

4. The approximation method of Log-rank test

$$\chi^2 = \sum_{g=1}^{k} \frac{\left(A_g - T_g\right)^2}{T_g} \tag{14.12}$$

is more conservative than the exact method. The general formula of the test statistic is

$$\chi^2 = \frac{\left[\Sigma w_i \left(d_{gi} - T_{gi}\right)\right]^2}{V_g} \tag{14.13}$$

where w_i is the weight, $w_i = 1$ for the log-rank test, while $w_i = n_i$ corresponding to the Breslow test. Because the Breslow test gives more weight to early time points than to late time points (n_i never increases with time), it is less sensitive than the log-rank test to differences between groups that occur at later points of time.

14.4   Application

14.4.1   Kaplan–Meier Procedure

SPSS procedure for Examples 14.1 and 14.3

1. **SPSS Data Set**

    Name "*group*" for group variable and name "*t*" for time variable. SPSS data set is shown in Fig. 14.3.

2. Procedure in SPSS Statistics

    (a) Click Analyze > Survival > Kaplan–Meier, as shown in Fig. 14.3.

    (b) Move the survival time variable [*t*] to the Time box, the variable [*status*] to the Status box. Click the button Define Event and enter "1" into the Single value box. Then move the variable [*group*] to the Factor box. Click Options and leave the Survival table(s). Tick the *Mean* and *median* survival checkboxes in the Statistics area and select the Survival and Hazard checkbox in the Plots area. Click Continue.

    (c) Click Compare Factor and select Log-rank and Breslow, click Continue and click OK.

3. Output results

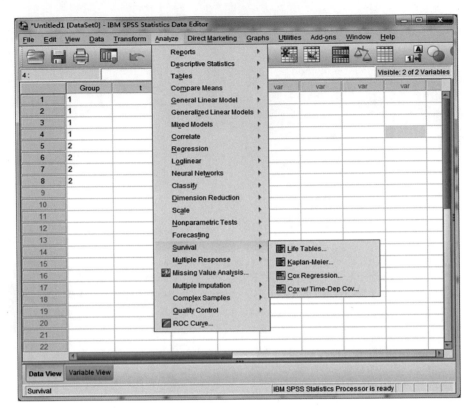

Fig. 14.3 Analyze → survival → Kaplan–Meier procedure

Fig. 14.4 Case processing
summary output

group	Total N	N of Events	Censored	
			N	Percent
1	11	8	3	27.3%
2	9	9		0.0%
Overall	20	17	3	15.0%

(a) Case processing summary: it includes group, total N, N of events, censored N, and censored percent (as shown in Fig. 14.4).

(b) Survival Table: It includes group, Time, Status, and Cumulative Proportion Surviving at the Time Estimate, *Std. Error*, N of Cumulative Events, and N of Remaining Cases (Fig. 14.5).

Survival Table

group		Time	Status	Cumulative Proportion Surviving at the Time		N of Cumulative Events	N of Remaining Cases
				Estimate	Std. Error		
1	1	5.000	1	.909	.087	1	10
	2	7.000	0	.	.	1	9
	3	13.000	1	.	.	2	8
	4	13.000	1	.707	.143	3	7
	5	23.000	1	.606	.154	4	6
	6	30.000	1	.505	.158	5	5
	7	30.000	0	.	.	5	4
	8	38.000	1	.379	.161	6	3
	9	42.000	1	.	.	7	2
	10	42.000	1	.126	.116	8	1
	11	45.000	0	.	.	8	0
2	1	1.000	1	.889	.105	1	8
	2	3.000	1	.	.	2	7
	3	3.000	1	.667	.157	3	6
	4	7.000	1	.556	.166	4	5
	5	10.000	1	.444	.166	5	4
	6	15.000	1	.	.	6	3
	7	15.000	1	.222	.139	7	2
	8	23.000	1	.111	.105	8	1
	9	30.000	1	.000	.000	9	0

Fig. 14.5 Survival table output

group	Mean[a]				Median			
	Estimate	Std. Error	95% Confidence Interval		Estimate	Std. Error	95% Confidence Interval	
			Lower Bound	Upper Bound			Lower Bound	Upper Bound
1	29.520	4.352	20.989	38.051	38.000	10.645	17.135	58.865
2	11.889	3.281	5.459	18.319	10.000	4.472	1.235	18.765
Overall	21.347	3.367	14.747	27.947	15.000	5.341	4.532	25.468

a. Estimation is limited to the largest survival time if it is censored

Fig. 14.6 *Means and medians* for survival time

Fig. 14.7 Output result of Log-rank test

Overall Comparisons

	Chi-Square	df	Sig.
Log-rank (Mantel-Cox)	7.628	1	.006
Breslow (Generalized Wilcoxon)	6.547	1	.011

Test of equality of survival distributions for the different levels of group.

(c) Means and medians for survival time: it includes group, *Mean (Estimate, Std. Error,* and 95% *Confidence Interval), Median (Estimate, Std. Error,* and 95% *Confidence Interval)* (shown in Fig. 14.6).

(d) The survival curve and hazard curve are shown in Fig. 14.1a, b.

(e) Overall Comparisons: It includes Chi-Square value, *df,* and *P* value (*Sig.*) in Log-rank test and Breslow test (shown in Fig. 14.7).

14.4.2 Life Tables Procedure

SPSS Procedure of Example 14.2

1. SPSS Data Set

   Set up a frequency variable called "*freq,*" name "*time*" for time variable, and name "*status*" for the status variable.

2. SPSS Procedure

   (a) Click weight cases in the menu of Data, click Weight cases by Analyze button, and move variable [*freq*] to the box below it. Click OK, and the dialogue box will be closed.

   Click Survival in the menu of Analyze and click Life tables, and you will be presented with the Life Tables dialogue box.

   (b) Move variable [*time*] to Time box, and enter 0–10 by 1 in the box below [*Display Time Intervals*]. Click variable [*status*] and click Define Event button, and enter "1" into the single value box. Click Options, and leave the Survival and Hazard checkbox in the Plots area. Click Continue, and you will be returned to the main dialogue box and then click OK.

3. Output results

   (a) Life Table: It includes Interval Start Time, Number Entering Interval, Number Withdrawing during Interval, Number Exposed to Risk, Number of Terminal Events, Proportion Terminating, Proportion Surviving, Cumulative Proportion Surviving at the End of Interval, *Std. Error* of Cumulative Proportion Surviving at the end of Interval, Probability Density, *Std. Error* of Probability Density, Hazard Rate, and *Std. Error* of Hazard Rate (as shown in Fig. 14.8).

   (b) The survival curve and hazard curve are shown in Fig. 14.2a, b.

Chapter Summary

1. Survival analysis is a class of statistical methods for studying the occurrence and timing of events. The end-point events include death, the effect of a treatment, relapse of diseases, and so on. Survival analysis is used to estimate or compare survival curves, explore related factors, and predict survival.

2. Kaplan–Meier method and life table method are two nonparametric methods to estimate the survival curve of survival data. Kaplan–Meier method is used for

Life Table[a]

Interval Start Time	Number Entering Interval	Number Withdrawing during Interval	Number Exposed to Risk	Number of Terminal Events	Proportion Terminating	Proportion Surviving	Cumulative Proportion Surviving at End of Interval	Std.Error of Cumulative Proportion Surviving at End of Interval	Probability Density	Std.Error of Probability Density	Hazard Rate	Std. Error of Hazard Rate
0	374	0	374.000	90	.24	.76	.76	.02	.241	.022	.27	.03
1	284	0	284.000	76	.27	.73	.56	.03	.203	.021	.31	.04
2	208	0	208.000	51	.25	.75	.42	.03	.136	.018	.28	.04
3	157	12	151.000	25	.17	.83	.35	.02	.070	.013	.18	.04
4	120	5	117.500	20	.17	.83	.29	.02	.060	.013	.19	.04
5	95	9	90.500	7	.08	.92	.27	.02	.022	.008	.08	.03
6	79	9	74.500	4	.05	.95	.25	.02	.014	.007	.06	.03
7	66	3	64.500	1	.02	.98	.25	.02	.004	.004	.02	.02
8	62	5	59.500	3	.05	.95	.24	.02	.013	.007	.05	.03
9	54	5	51.500	2	.04	.96	.23	.02	.009	.006	.04	.03
10	47	47	23.500	0	.00	1.00	.23	.02	.000	.000	.00	.00

a. The *median* survival time is 2.41

Fig. 14.8 Output result of survival rate in life table

Table 14.5 Survival analysis methods and SPSS procedures

Analytical purposes	Univariate analysis and SPSS procedure	Multivariate analysis and SPSS procedure
Estimating survival functions	Kaplan–Meier method (Kaplan–Meier procedure) Life table method (life tables procedure)	Proportional hazards model (cox regression)
Comparing survival curves	Log-rank test (Kaplan–Meier procedure)	Proportional hazards model (cox regression)
Analysis of influencing factors	Log-rank test (Kaplan–Meier procedure)	Proportional hazards model (cox regression)

small/large-sized not grouped data; life table method is used when data are grouped from a large sample. Both methods calculate the cumulative survival rate based on the product of the conditional probability of survival.

3. Log-rank test is a nonparametric method used to compare two or more survival curves; it is widely used because it allows overall comparison of survival curves.

4. Survival analysis can be carried out easily with many statistical computer packages such as SPSS software. Table 14.5 lists different survival analysis methods for various analytical purposes and their corresponding SPSS procedures.

Chapter 15
Cox Regression

Mingqin Cao

Objectives

Cox regression is a popular model used for analyzing survival data. The objective of this chapter is to study the general form of Cox regression and its characteristics, concepts of hazard ratio, and proportional hazard assumption, as well as the estimation and interpretation of regression parameters. The process of establishing a Cox regression model is carried out by SPSS software.

Key Concepts

Cox regression; Baseline hazard function; Hazard ratio; Proportional hazard assumption

15.1 Introduction

In Chap. 14, the methods of description and statistical inference were introduced for survival data, but only for single-factor analysis. In this chapter, a popular multivariate regression method for survival data, which is known as the Cox proportional hazards regression model (abbreviated to Cox PH regression or Cox regression), will be introduced. It was first proposed by a British biostatistician D. R. Cox in 1972 and widely used in medical and clinical research afterwards. Cox regression is similar to linear regression and logistic regression that it can screen factors related to the outcome. The difference is that Cox regression can be used for time-to-event outcome measures while linear regression and logistic regression can be used for continuous and classified outcome measures, respectively.

M. Cao (✉)

School of Public Health, Xingjiang Medical University, Urumqi, China

© Zhengzhou University Press 2024

X. Guo, F. Xue (eds.), *Textbook of Medical Statistics*,

https://doi.org/10.1007/978-981-99-7390-3_15

15.2 Introduction to Cox Regression

15.2.1 Data Structure

Cox proportional hazards regression is the most commonly used model for analyzing survival data. The data structure of Cox regression is similar to that of multivariate linear regression or logistic regression, which is given in Table 15.1.

In the data structure table, each row represents a single individual and each column represents a single independent variable or dependent variable. The first column of Table 15.1 represents the serial number of the study objects. The following p columns shows the values of a set of explanatory variables of interest (X_1, X_2, ..., X_p). The last two columns show the information of outcome measures: T is a continuous variable which gives the observed survival time of each object, and Y is a dichotomous variable which indicates the status of censorship ($Y = 1$, terminal event occurs; $Y = 0$, censored value, terminal event absent).

There are no specific requirements for the type of independent variables in Cox regression analysis. The explanatory variable X_i can be either continuous or discrete variable. For example, X_i can be age, gender, nationality, anemia status, etc. Age (years) is a quantitative variable recorded as numerical values. Gender is a binary variable usually recorded as 1 (male) or 2 (female). Nationality (such as Han, Uygur, Kazak, and other minorities) is a polytomous variable usually recorded from 1 to 4, but should be transformed into three dummy variables when fitting the regression model. Anemia status (such as normal, mild anemia, moderate anemia, severe anemia, etc.) is an ordered categorical variable usually ranked from 1 to 4 according to anemia degree.

There are two dependent variables: survival time T and outcome status Y when fitting Cox regression model. T is a continuous variable representing the length of time from the beginning of study to the occurrence of failure event or being censored. Several reasons may account for being censored: the failure event or the event of interest does not occur until the end of the study; loss to follow-up; or withdrawal before the end of the study. Y is a binary variable with value 1 or 0, $Y = 1$ means the failure event occurs while $Y = 0$ means being censored.

Example 15.1 To study whether a drug can improve the prognosis of leukemia patients and prolong their remission time, 42 patients who met clinical diagnostic criteria of leukemia were randomly assigned to two groups: one group received a certain treatment; the other group received placebo. In this example, going out of

Table 15.1 Data structure of the Cox regression

Number	X_1	X_2	...	X_p	T (time)	Y (outcome)
1	a_{11}	a_{12}	...	a_{1p}	t_1	y_1
2	a_{21}	a_{22}	...	a_{2p}	t_2	y_2
...	...	...	...	...	...	...
n	a_{n1}	a_{n2}	...	a_{np}	t_n	y_n

remission is a failure event, and remission duration for each patient was recorded in weeks. Considering the white blood cell count (WBC) may affect the efficacy of treatment, each patient's log WBC is measured before treatment. The data is shown in Table 15.2 (data from Freireich et al. Blood, 1963). Try to analyze whether the treatment can improve the prognosis and prolong the remission duration of leukemia patients.

The study was a clinical research, and the purpose was to compare the treatment effects between treatment group and placebo group. For 42 leukemia patients, outcomes were measured with remission duration and remission status. It is well known that the WBC is usually considered as an important predictor of survival in leukemia patients: the higher the WBC, the worse the prognosis. Thus, comparison of the effects between the two treatment groups needs to consider the possible confounding effect of logWBC.

There are two independent variables: treatment and logWBC. Treatment is a binary variable recorded as 1 or 2 (1 = treatment group, 2 = placebo group). There are two dependent variables: remission duration and remission status. The remission status is a dichotomous variable recorded as 1or 0 (1 = going out of remission or failure event, 0 = in remission or censored status). As is given in Table 15.3, the

Table 15.2 The raw observations about 42 leukemia patients after treatment

Treatment ($n = 21$)			Placebo ($n = 21$)		
No.	logWBC	Remission time (weeks)	No.	logWBC	Remission time (weeks)
1	2.31	6	22	2.80	1
2	4.06	6	23	5.00	1
3	3.28	6	24	4.91	2
4	4.43	7	25	4.48	2
5	2.96	10	26	4.01	3
6	2.88	13	27	4.36	4
7	3.60	16	28	2.42	4
8	2.32	22	29	3.49	5
9	2.57	23	30	3.97	5
10	3.20	6+	31	3.52	8
11	2.80	9+	32	3.05	8
12	2.70	10+	33	2.32	8
13	2.60	11+	34	3.26	8
14	2.16	17+	35	3.49	11
15	2.05	19+	36	2.12	11
16	2.01	20+	37	1.50	12
17	1.78	25+	38	3.06	12
18	2.20	32+	39	2.30	15
19	2.53	32+	40	2.95	17
20	1.47	34+	41	2.73	22
21	1.45	35+	42	1.97	23

+ Indicates censored data, logWBC is logarithm transformation of WBC in order to reduce variation of data

Table 15.3 Data structure of survival analysis at Example 15.1

No.	Groups	Log WBC	Remission time (weeks)	Remission status
1	1	2.31	6	1
2	1	4.06	6	1
3	1	3.28	6	1
4	1	4.43	7	1
5	1	2.96	10	1
6	1	2.88	13	1
7	1	3.60	16	1
8	1	2.32	22	1
9	1	2.57	23	1
10	1	3.20	6	0
11	1	2.80	9	0
12	1	2.70	10	0
13	1	2.60	11	0
14	1	2.16	17	0
15	1	2.05	19	0
16	1	2.01	20	0
17	1	1.78	25	0
18	1	2.20	32	0
19	1	2.53	32	0
20	1	1.47	34	0
21	1	1.45	35	0
22	2	2.80	1	1
23	2	5.00	1	1
24	2	4.91	2	1
25	2	4.48	2	1
26	2	4.01	3	1
27	2	4.36	4	1
28	2	2.42	4	1
29	2	3.49	5	1
30	2	3.97	5	1
31	2	3.52	8	1
32	2	3.05	8	1
33	2	2.32	8	1
34	2	3.26	8	1
35	2	3.49	11	1
36	2	2.12	11	1
37	2	1.50	12	1
38	2	3.06	12	1
39	2	2.30	15	1
40	2	2.95	17	1
41	2	2.73	22	1
42	2	1.97	23	1

basic data structure includes 42 rows (42 patients' observations) and 5 columns (Patients ID, two independent variables, and two dependent variables) in survival analysis of Example 15.1.

15.2.2 The General Form of Cox Regression

Cox regression model is generally written in terms of the hazard function model. This model gives an expression for the hazard at time t for individual with a given specification of a set of explanatory variables ($X_1, X_2, ..., X_p$). Assume $h(t,X)$ is the hazard function at time t with X representing a collection of explanatory variables, the link function is an exponential function, the general form of Cox regression model is as follows:

$$h(t,X) = h_0(t)\exp\left(\beta_1 X_1 + \beta_2 X_2 + ... + \beta_p X_p\right).$$

(15.1)

In this formula, $h_0(t)$ is the baseline hazard function, which represents the risk at time t when all the independent variables are equal to zero. $\beta_i (i = 1, 2, ..., p)$ is the partial regression coefficient of independent variable X_i. Exp() is the exponential expression e to the liner sum of $\beta_i X_i$, which does not involve t. That is, independent variables are independent with time.

The baseline hazard function, $h_0(t)$, is an unspecified function, which involves time t but no independent variables. Without information of $h_0(t)$, it is still possible to estimate every regression coefficient in the exponential part of the Cox model. Therefore, the Cox regression model is also called semiparametric model.

15.2.3 Why Cox Model is Popular

Censored values are often seen in cohort or follow-up studies, and multivariate analysis of survival data becomes more important in medical research. Cox regression model is so widely used in survival analysis when dealing with multiple explanatory variables.

One of the reasons why Cox model is so popular is that Cox model is a "robust" model, so the results of Cox model will closely approximate the results of the correct parametric model.

Another appealing property of Cox model is that the specific form of Cox model gives the hazard function as a product of a baseline hazard and an exponential expression involving independent variables, which ensures the fitted model will always give non-negative estimated hazard. We want such non-negative estimates because, by definition, the values of any hazard function must range between 0 and $+\infty$.

   The third reason about the popularity of Cox model is that it is semiparametric. Even though the baseline hazard part of model is unknown, the partial regression coefficients, β_i, can still be estimated and explained. Estimates of regression coefficient will be used to assess the effect of explanatory variables of interest. The measure of effect is called hazard ratio (*HR*), which is similar to the relative risk (*RR*) in epidemiological interpretation.

   One last point about the popularity of Cox model is that it is preferred over the logistic model when survival time information is available and there is censoring. That is, the Cox model can use more information of survival time and censoring, but the logistic model only considers a (0, 1) outcome and ignores survival time and censoring.

15.3   Principles of Cox Regression

15.3.1   The Hazard Ratio (HR)

In general, a hazard ratio (*HR*) is defined as the hazard for an individual divided by the hazard for another individual given the same time t. Assume $X^* = \left(X_1^*, X_2^*, \ldots, X_p^* \right)$ is expressed as the set of predictors for one individual, and $X = (X_1, X_2, \ldots, X_p)$ is expressed as the set of predictors for another individual. At time t, the hazard ratio of the two individuals is expressed as

$$HR = \frac{h(t,X^*)}{h(t,X)} = \frac{h_0(t)\exp\left(\beta_1 X_1^* + \beta_2 X_2^* + \ldots + \beta_p X_p^*\right)}{h_0(t)\exp\left(\beta_1 X_1 + \beta_2 X_2 + \ldots + \beta_p X_p\right)}. \tag{15.2}$$

   They have the same baseline hazard function, $h0(t)$, because $h0(t)$ is independent of explanatory variables. That is,

$$HR = \exp\left[\sum_{i=1}^{p} \beta_i \left(X_i^* - X_i \right) \right]. \tag{15.3}$$

   Assume that the failure event is death, $h(t,X)$ is the hazard function for death with predictors X at time t, and there are only one predictor X_1 ($X_1 = 1$ means the person has a certain exposure feature, and $X_1 = 0$ means the person has not this exposure feature), then *HR* is calculated as: $HR = \exp[\beta_1 \times (1 - 0)] = \exp \beta_1$ to compare exposed individual with non-exposed individual. If $\beta_1 > 0$, then $HR > 1$, meaning the person having exposure feature has larger hazard of death than that of the person with non-exposure feature, and the exposure feature is called risk factor. If $\beta_1 = 0$, then $HR = 1$, meaning the exposure factor is not associated with death. If $\beta_1 < 0$, then $HR < 1$, meaning the person having exposure feature has smaller hazard of death than that of the person with non-exposure feature, and the exposure feature is called protective factor.

Thus, $HR = \exp \beta_i$ or $\beta_i = \ln (HR)$ can well explain the relationship between exposure factor X_i and the hazard for outcome occurrence while X_i is a dichotomous variable with $X_i = 1$ meaning larger hazard and $X_i = 0$ meaning smaller hazard in clinical epidemiological study. Furthermore, there are a set of exposure variables $(X_1, X_2, \ldots, X_p)$, β_i is the regression coefficient of X_i, with $HR = \exp \beta_i$ considering the value of X_i increase one unit to X_i meanwhile the values of all other exposure variable are invariableness.

For example, we can do the Cox regression analysis of the data of Example 15.1 by SPSS software, the Cox regression model is as following:

$$h(t,X) = h_0(t)\exp(1.294 \times \text{groups} + 1.604 \times \log WBC)$$

The regression coefficient of group variable (treatment = 1, placebo = 2) was 1.294, which means the hazard ratio HR for going out of remission is $\exp(1.294) = 3.648$ when comparing placebo with treatment having logWBC controlled on the same value. The result shows that individual of placebo group had higher risk of deterioration than that of treatment group, or the treatment group have better efficacy of remission than the placebo group. Similarly, the regression coefficient of logWBC was 1.604, which means that the higher value of logWBC, the worse prognosis of patients, and higher value of logWBC is a risk factor of patients' prognosis.

15.3.2   Maximum Likelihood (ML) Estimates

The parameters of Cox regression are estimated by maximum likelihood (ML) estimates, which is similar to logistic regression model. The formula for the Cox model likelihood function is called partial likelihood function because the likelihood formula only considers probabilities for those subjects who fail, and does not consider probabilities for those subjects who are censored. Once the likelihood function is formed for given model, the next step for the computer is to maximize this function by the Newton-Raphson iteration method, which is computationally easier by statistical software.

15.3.3   Hypothesis Testing and Confidence Interval Estimation

Once the ML estimates are obtained, we are usually interested in carrying out statistical inferences on the estimates of regression coefficients. Assume b_i is the estimate of β_i, S_{bi} is the standard error of b_i, the Wald test is commonly used to make the hypothesis that whether the population regression coefficients, β_i, equals to 0. The formula of the Wald test is

$$\chi^2 = \frac{b_i}{S_{b_i}}, \quad v = 1. \tag{15.4}$$

The 95% confidence intervals for a regression coefficient is estimated as $b_i \pm 1.96 S_{b_i}$ considering the distribution of statistic is approximate to the normal distributions in a large sample size, and the 95% confidence interval for hazard ratio (HR) is estimated as $\exp\left(b_i \pm 1.96 S_{b_i}\right)$.

For example, the output of the Cox regression analysis for Example 15.1 is shown in Fig. 15.1 by SPSS software. We find the estimate of group variable is 1.294, its Wald test $\chi^2 = 1.294/0.422 = 9.399$, and the P value 0.002, which means the relationship is statistically significant between the explanatory variable group and survival outcome. The estimate of HR of group variable is $\exp(1.294)=3.648$, and the 95% confidence interval of HR of group is $\exp(1.294 \pm 1.96 \times 0.422)$, that is, the 95% CI is from 1.595 to 8.343.

15.3.4 The Meaning of the Proportional Hazard Assumption

Cox regression model needs to meet the proportional hazard (PH) assumption. The PH assumption requires that the HR is constant over time, or equivalently, that the hazard for one individual is proportional to the hazard for any other individual, where the proportionality constant is independent of time.

To explain the PH assumption, we consider the Cox regression model for the remission data of 42 leukemia patients involving the two variables: group and log-WBC. In this model, the estimate of hazard ratio comparing placebo group with treatment group while controlling for log WBC is computed by the formula

$$HR = \frac{h(t,group = 2, \log WBC)}{h(t,group = 1, \log WBC)} = \exp(1.294) = 3.648.$$

The value of HR is a constant of 3.648. Thus, the hazard for placebo is 3.648 times the hazard for the treatment group, and the value, 3.648, is the same regardless of time. If the Cox PH model is inappropriate, the time-dependent Cox model should be carried out.

Variables in the Equation

	B	SE	Wald	df	Sig.	Exp(B)	95.0% CI for Exp(B)	
							Lower	Upper
groups	1.294	.422	9.399	1	.002	3.648	1.595	8.343
logWBC	1.604	.329	23.732	1	.000	4.975	2.609	9.486

Fig. 15.1 Outcome of Cox regression analysis of Example 15.1

15.4   Application

We demonstrate how to carry out the Cox regression analysis using the remission data of Example 15.1 by SPSS software. There are 42 leukemia patients assigned into two groups with 21 patients in the placebo group and the other 21 patients in the treatment group. The logWBC of each patient was also obtained before treatment. There are two explanatory variables and censored data, so the Cox regression should be applied to analyze survival data with multiple explanatory variables.

15.4.1   Building a SPSS Data File

The data structure for survival analysis is provided in Table 15.3: the 'group' variable is coded as 1 or 2 (group = 1 for the treatment group, group = 2 for the placebo group); logWBC is input as numeric value; the variable of weeks is continuous value of remission time; the variable of output is outcome status, coded as 0 or 1 (output= 1 for going out of remission or being worse, output = 0 for the censored data.

15.4.2   Cox Regression Model by SPSS

The main process to perform the Cox regression of Example 15.1 is
  Navigate to Analyze → Survival → Cox Regression, then select 'weeks' for Time and 'output' for Status → group, logWBC → select to Covariate → Method→ Enter → Options → OK.
  Step by step process:

1. Analyze → Survival → Cox Regression, Enter the Cox regression analysis model, as shown in Fig. 15.2.
2. In Cox Regression windows, select "remission time [weeks]" to Time, select outcome "output" to Status, "Define Event" defined single value of 1, select "treatment group[group]" and "white blood cell count[logWBC]" to Covariate, Method select "Enter". Click "Options", the Options window of Cox Regression will appear. Check "CI for exp(B) 95%" under "Model Statistics" and click the "Continue" button. Back to the Cox Regression window, click the "OK" button.

15.4.3   Main Output Results

The results of the Cox regression models by Enter method are shown in Figs. 15.3 and 15.4. There are 30 patients of failure event and 12 patients of censored values, the percent of censored number is 28.6% in total number.

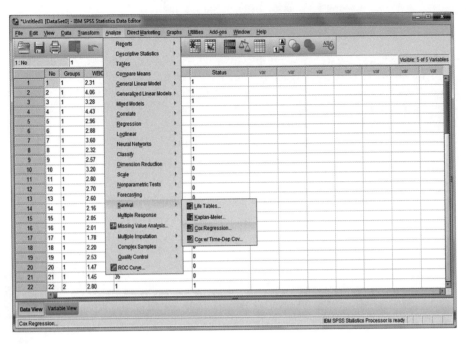

Fig. 15.2 Enter the Cox Regression model

Case Processing Summary

		N	Percent
Cases available in analysis	Event[a]	30	71.4%
	Censored	12	28.6%
	Total	42	100.0%
Cases dropped	Cases with missing values	0	0.0%
	Cases with negative time	0	0.0%
	Censored cases before the earliest event in a stratum	0	0.0%
	Total	0	0.0%
Total		42	100.0%

a. Dependent Variable: remisson time

Fig. 15.3 Case processing summary of remission data

This Cox model is statistically significant ($P < 0.001$), and two explanatory variables: group ($P = 0.002$) and logWBC ($P < 0.001$) are also statistically significant in the model. The regression coefficient B, the standard error SE, the Wald test, the

Block 0: Beginning Block

Omnibus
Tests of
Model
Coefficients

-2 Log Likelihood
187.970

Block 1: Method = Enter

Omnibus Tests of Model Coefficients[a]

-2 Log Likelihood	Overall (score)			Change From Previous Step			Change From Previous Block		
	Chi-square	df	Sig.	Chi-square	df	Sig.	Chi-square	df	Sig.
144.559	42.938	2	.000	43.412	2	.000	43.412	2	.000

a. Beginning Block Number 1. Method = Enter

Variables in the Equation

	B	SE	Wald	df	Sig.	Exp(B)	95.0% CI for Exp(B)	
							Lower	Upper
groups	1.294	.422	9.399	1	.002	3.648	1.595	8.343
logWBC	1.604	.329	23.732	1	.000	4.975	2.609	9.486

Fig. 15.4 The main output of the Cox regression of remission data

P value Sig., the HR estimate Exp(B), and the 95% confidence interval for Exp(B) of two explanatory variables are all shown in Fig. 15.4. The regression coefficient of group is 1.294, $P = 0.002$, the HR for group is 3.648, and the 95% confidence interval is (1.595, 8.343). The regression coefficient of logWBC is 1.604, $P < 0.001$, the HR for logWBC is 4.975, and the 95% confidence interval is (2.609, 9.486). The Cox regression model is written as:

$$h(t,X) = h_0(t)\exp(1.294 \times group + 1.604 \times \log WBC)$$

15.4.4 Conclusion

The remission time of leukemia patients is influenced by the treatment group and patient's logWBC. Drug treatment, compared with placebo, can make the patient's remission time longer; the leukocyte count also affect the treatment outcome of patients, and the higher level of leukocyte count, the worse of the patient's prognosis. Therefore, giving treatment and controlling the level of leukocyte cells would alleviate the disease and prolong the remission time.

Chapter Summary
1. Cox regression model is commonly used for analyzing survival data with multiple explanatory variables. There are two outcome variables: survival time *t* (continuous value) and survival status with 0 or 1 (1 = failure event occurrence, 0 = censored).

2. The general form of Cox regression model is:

   $h(t, X) = h_0(t) \exp(\beta_1 X_1 + \beta_2 X_2 + \ldots + \beta_p X_p)$. The baseline hazard function, $h_0(t)$, is unknown or uncertain, so that the Cox regression model is known as semiparametric regression model.

3. The hazard ratio (HR) is a ratio that the hazard function for one individual divided by the hazard function for another individual. The relationship between HR and regression coefficient β_i in the Cox regression is $HR = \exp(\beta)$ or $\beta = \ln(HR)$, which can be explained the same way as the OR in logistic regression.

4. The PH assumption is that the HR is a constant regardless of time, or the effect of independent variables is independent of time.